Mechanical Link

Mechanical Link

Fundamental Principles, Theory, and Practice Following an Osteopathic Approach

Paul Chauffour, D.O., M.R.O.
Eric Prat, D.O., M.R.O.

Translated by Monique Bureau, P.T., D.O.

Foreword by Jean-Pierre Barral, D.O.

UI Enterprises
Palm Beach Gardens, Florida

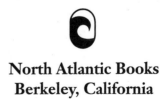

North Atlantic Books
Berkeley, California

Published by
North Atlantic Books   UI Enterprises
P.O. Box 12327   11211 Prosperity Farms Road
Berkeley, California 94712   Palm Beach Gardens, Florida 33410

Cover and book design by Jennifer Dunn
Printed in the United States of America

Mechanical Link: Fundamental Principles, Theory, and Practice Following an Osteopathic Approach is sponsored by the Society for the Study of Native Arts and Sciences, a nonprofit educational corporation whose goals are to develop an educational and crosscultural perspective linking various scientific, social, and artistic fields; to nurture a holistic view of arts, sciences, humanities, and healing; and to publish and distribute literature on the relationship of mind, body, and nature.

North Atlantic Books are available through most bookstores. To contact North Atlantic directly, call (800) 337-2665 or visit our website at www.northatlanticbooks.com.

Substantial discounts on bulk quantities of North Atlantic books are available to corporations, professional associations, and other organizations. For details and discount information, contact the special sales department at North Atlantic Books.

Library of Congress Cataloging-in-Publication Data
Chauffour, Paul.
    [Lien mecanique. English]
    Mechanical link : fundamental principles, theory, and practice following an osteopathic approach / by Paul Chauffour and Eric Prat ; translated by Monique Bureau.
        p. ; cm.
Includes bibliographical references and index.
    ISBN 1-55643-427-8 (hardcover)
    1. Osteopathic medicine. 2. Osteopathic orthopedics.
    [DNLM: 1. Manipulation, Osteopathic. WB 535 C496L 2002a] I. Prat, Eric, 1959– II. Title.
    RZ342 .C475 2002
    615.5'33—dc21
                                                    2002151202

1 2 3 4 5 6 7 / 06 05 04 03 02

This book is dedicated to many people:

our patients, the reason for this work;

our Mechanical Link students, for whom this work has finally been completed;

the people close to us that made this work possible, especially Sylvie;

the readers, who we hope will find this work to be thought-provoking.

We would also like to thank the CIDO and The Upledger Institute for their confidence in us and for the promotion of *Mechanical Link* in Europe and the United States and Canada.

Contents

CHAPTER 12

The Vascular Unit   *119*

CHAPTER 13

The Cephalic Unit   *131*

List of Figures

Foreword

Osteopathy and physical therapy are highly regarded throughout Europe, and Paul Chauffour is renowned as one of our first pioneers. He has had a major influence on the landscape of healthcare with his original form of therapy based on subtle manual listening.

Starting from any point on the body, Paul is able to use his Mechanical Link method to determine, quickly and precisely, which parts need to be helped. The techniques are performed with very little recoil in order to stimulate the auto-corrective action of the organism. In this way they never force change upon the body but instead create the opportunity for the body to heal itself.

Paul is an artist, and his method is so gentle it can be applied as successfully to the newborn baby as the elderly. He is an excellent practitioner and a good man, and it shows whenever he treats a patient or teaches a student.

I am honored to call Paul a friend. And I warmly encourage every manual therapist to read his book and learn from him.

— Jean-Pierre Barral, DO

Introduction

Twenty years ago we formulated the elements that were to become *Mechanical Link*. At that time we had no idea how those concepts would develop and how far they would take us. In this book, we invite readers to share the results of our research, experience, and clinical practice.

Mechanical Link could be presented as an osteopathic method, at the same time traditional and modern, empirical and scientific, global and analytical. *Traditional*, because our work is based on the essential principles of A.T. Still, principles that we think deserve to be continually deepened; *modern*, because our manual approach has evolved toward a technique that is very innovative and sophisticated while still adhering to fundamental concepts such as that "the structure governs the function," that "the role of the artery is absolute," or "research for the cause." We adhere to these while at the same time presenting a new way to approach the osteopathic lesion.

Mechanical Link is *empirical* because our work is most of all inspired by our experience in our daily practice. It is also *scientific* because we have attempted to maintain rigor and reproducibility, which is indispensable for medical research. Mechanical Link, inspired by personal research and observation, takes into consideration the knowledge of embryology, anatomy, and physiology. These areas will be reviewed in this text to enable the greatest understanding of our approach.

Our work is *global* because, contrary to systemic medicine, we consider the human body to be formed by functional units that are interdependent and biomechanically linked to one another. Furthermore, the concept of Mechanical Link is *analytical* because we seek to discover all the possible lesions in each anatomic territory. The concept of *total lesion* necessitates the overall and complete evaluation of the body. The concept of *primary lesion* involves distilling the results of this analysis to determine the points of fixation to be treated.

Through this work we endeavor to clearly present the key elements of the Mechanical Link perspective. As with most areas of study, the reading of a text is not enough to insure the correct practice of the techniques. We strongly recommend that those who wish to incorporate Mechanical Link into their practice should undertake rigorous training.

A Brief History of Osteopathy

Andrew Taylor Still, a medical doctor and surgeon, pioneered the field of osteopathy in 1874. Disenchanted with medicine, he had stopped prescribing medication and performing surgeries. Instead he began treating his patients manually, developing a series of osteopathic principles—including "structure governs function both locally and globally"—that we still follow today.

Dr. Still is widely considered the first physician to treat each patient as a whole while searching for the causes of dysfunction rather than treating symptoms. His dedication was rewarded with great success, restoring the dynamic equilibrium of the structures and the quality of natural functioning to the individual. He established the first college of osteopathy in Kirksville, Missouri, in 1892.

Early in the 20th century, William Garner Sutherland, D.O., who had been trained by Dr. Still, formed the concept of the primary respiratory mechanism that he used to develop the field of cranial osteopathy. Yet he continued to insist that his students treat each patient with a global perspective, not limiting themselves exclusively to the use of cranial osteopathy.

In 1917 osteopathy took root in Europe thanks to another one of Dr. Still's students: John Martin Littlejohn, D.O., who founded the British School of Osteopathy. He also discovered the lines of gravity used so effectively in manual therapies such as Mechanical Link. While osteopathy in America continued to evolve around the practice of allopathic medicine, European osteopathy progressed toward a biodynamic approach.

This branch relies more on the art of palpation and refined manual therapeutic techniques.

Today there are many colleges of osteopathy around the world. The first French osteopathic colleges in particular formed the roots for institutions in countries across Europe. Yet unlike American osteopaths who are trained as medical doctors, osteopaths outside the U.S. are required to take a 5- to 6-year doctorate program in osteopathic manual practice. They must also conduct extensive clinical research and produce a thesis to earn their doctorates.

Today French osteopathy remains a renowned and highly respected field. Its rich tradition has been expanded and refined in several key areas, including that of the Mechanical Link approach developed by Paul Chauffour, D.O.

—Monique Bureau, P.T., D.O.

CHAPTER 1

Embryology and Histology of Connective Tissue

The Importance of a Review of Embryology

Throughout existence the past has influenced the present, and each particular moment includes the ones that preceded it. The study of a living structure would not be complete if we looked at only its anatomy and physiology. We also have to be interested in its history. In the case of the human body, we must study its embryology. In the context of this short chapter we will not review the entirety of embryology, as many books have been written on this subject, and if interested in a deeper review, the reader is encouraged to consult these adjunctive texts. However, it is important that we focus on a few key points of embryology that will assist in explaining our osteopathic approach.

Mechanical Link is a manual therapeutic method that analyzes a range of anatomical structures: joints, fasciae, bones, arteries, derma, etc. Fundamental to our osteopathic practice is the recognition that all of these elements come from the same embryological inheritance, the *mesoblast*.

The Mesoblast as a Link

There are three primitive sheaths or germ layers of the embryo that give birth to all tissues and organs. These sheaths are in place by the third

Figure 1

The Mesoblast

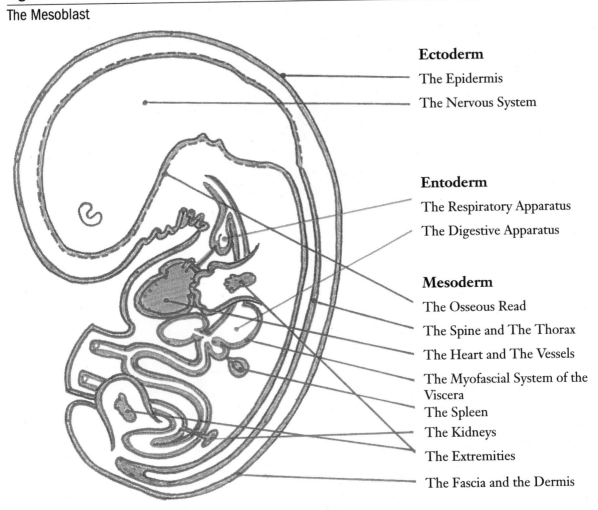

Ectoderm

The Epidermis

The Nervous System

Entoderm

The Respiratory Apparatus

The Digestive Apparatus

Mesoderm

The Osseous Read

The Spine and The Thorax

The Heart and The Vessels

The Myofascial System of the Viscera

The Spleen

The Kidneys

The Extremities

The Fascia and the Dermis

week of human development. This phase is called *gastrulation*, and the three sheaths are described as:

- the *endoblast* or internal sheath;
- the *ectoblast* or external sheath;
- the *mesoblast* or the middle sheath.

The appearance of the mesoblast corresponds to the beginning of the embryogenesis: the formation of the embryo. Its intermediary position between the two other sheaths already implies that it is a *link*. As we will see, this is very important.

The Mechanical Similarity of All Connective Tissues

Found everywhere in the body—connecting and unifying—the connective tissue can be considered the organic cement of human tectonic architecture. It ensures the structural cohesion of all the different functional units of the organism, and is always an intimate part of it. Derived from the mesoblast, the embryonic connective tissue (the mesenchyme) gives birth to all the various types of adult connective tissue.

Here are the types of connective tissue in order of least to most dense:
- the blood and lymph—liquid connective tissue;
- the loose connective tissue—adipose, reticular, areolar;
- the dense and elastic connective tissue;
- the cartilage;
- the bone.

No matter what its form or function, the connective tissue consists of three parts.

1. The cells, which all originate from the mesenchyme, will later specialize
- depending on their function:
- erythrocytes, leucocytes, and thrombocytes of the vascular tissue;
- adipocytes of the adipose tissue;
- fibroblasts of the fascial tissue;
- chondrocytes of the cartilage;
- osteocytes of the bone.

2. There are three distinct types of fibers that make up the structure of the connective tissue. The variable proportions of these three types of fibers create a different biomechanical characteristic that is specific to the type of connective tissue that it forms. Each will differ in degree of flexibility, elasticity, or resistance of these elements.
- The reticular fibers take the form of a trellis and form a ramified (branching) network of organic tissue.
- The elastic fibers are very ductile (flexible).
- The collagen fibers are very resistant and organized into spindles.

3. The fundamental substance constitutes the metabolic environment in which all the cells and connective tissues soak and develop. It can be of a liquid, gelatinous, or solid consistency.

Because they all contain the same three elements, we can say that all these diverse systems, such as the osteoarticular system, the fascial system, and the vascular system, which seem to be anatomically very different, are embryologically homogenous. In addition, this similar inheritance creates a physical (structure) and a physiological (function) continuity.

- The osseous tissue provides insertions for the fasciae, and there the blood cells originate.
- The fascial tissue envelops and supports the osteoarticular system, as well as the vessels.
- The blood tissue irrigates all connective tissue mentioned above, with the exception of avascular areas of the articular cartilage.

The Myofascial System

Toward the end of the period of gastrulation, the paraxial mesoblast segments into forty-four pairs of somites. This is the origin of the somatic organization in the human body.

The skeletal muscles originate from the myotomes of the somites. They develop jointly with the fasciae, which originate from the sclerotome of the same somites. We can therefore consider the muscular system and the fascial system as being the active and passive elements, respectively, of the same connective tissue entity.

The heart, which belongs at the same time to the muscular and to the vascular system, is a striated muscle. It is an interesting muscle because its functioning is entirely automatic. Embryologically, its development takes place in conjunction with the development of the vascular system and becomes the principal motor of that system. The pericardia fascia is formed from the same mesenchymatous cells as the myocardium carriage that it envelops.

The smooth muscles, which insure the contraction of the viscera, also originate from this splanchnic (visceral) mesoblast. Their growth is closely related to the growth of the primitive intestine and its derivatives. The primitive intestine and its derivatives originate from the endoblast.

The pleura and the peritoneum, of mesoblastic origin, are the serous sheaths or sacs, which envelop the pulmonary and the digestive apparatus. Their expansions form the ligamentous system and the connective girdle around the organs and viscera. Therefore, we can see that right from the beginning the myofascial system is present during the intrinsic and extrinsic development of the viscero-organic unit. Because of this, it provides a structural cohesion. In general, the organs and viscera are from the parenchyma and epithelium of endoblastic origin, while all surrounding connective tissue and smooth muscle derive from the adjacent mesoblast.

Embryologically, the skin deserves special consideration because the derma is a functional fascial unit that also originates from the mesoblastic connective tissue. Only the superficial layer of the epidermis and its annexes (the glands, hair, and nails) are from the ectoblast. The derma develops from the mesenchymatous cells of the somites and forms following the particular segmentation of the dermatomes. In Mechanical Link we consider the derma and the superficialis fasciae, which it covers, as a connective functional unit. We will systematically integrate this functional unit into the osteopathic examination and treatment.

The cranial and spinal dura mater (with its expansions—the falx cerebri, the tentorium cerebelli, and the falx cerebelli) constitutes the most external and most resistant of the three meninges. The pia mater and the arachnoid originate, as does the nervous system, from the ectoblast. The dura mater originates from the mesoderm, just as do all other elements of the myofascial system. Therefore, the dura mater is a connective structure, which we must take into consideration. The sheaths of the peripheral nervous system (the girdles around the nerves) also originate from the mesoderm. They are anatomically connected to the dura mater at the vertebral foramen where they exit.

The Osseous System

The entire osteoarticular system develops from the mesoblast. The skeleton of the human embryo first has a rough form of connective tissue made of fibrous membranes and hyaline cartilage. The mesenchymatous cells will become the osteoblasts, which then function to progressively ossify this connective tissue. We distinguish a *membranous ossification*, which is mostly of the cranial vault—the maxillary and the clavicle—from the *endochondral ossification* of the other elements of the skeleton.

The osseous head develops from a membranous model at the vault, and a cartilaginous model at the base. Some bones, such as the temporal bone, are part of both of these osteogenic models. We can find dissociated lesions between the squama (membranous ossification) and the mastoid (endochondral ossification). An example of a dissociated lesion would be an external rotation of the squama (the temporal bone is anterior) and an anterior mastoid (the temporal bone is posterior).

The ossification centers of the cranial vault (membranous neurocranium) appear during the ninth week of the embryologic development. They will form the frontal, the parietal, and occipital ossification centers. We can see their importance in the tectonic architecture of the cranium. The anterior fontanel, which ossifies during the second year of life, represents the keystone of the vault of the calvaria (skull). We often find the bregma implicated in the lesional organization of the cranium.

A cartilaginous model precedes the osteogenesis of the cranial base. The development of the cranial floor is organized around a system of beams that converge toward the sella turcica of the sphenoid. These beams must be considered as part of the intraosseous line of force of the cranium. We will demonstrate the importance of this in our discussion of the osteopathic treatment and examination of the lines of force of the osseous head (Chapter 10).

The teeth, except for the enamel that covers the dental crown, also are of mesoblastic origin. The dentin, which constitutes the body of the tooth, is like a bone. It is a calcified connective tissue. The cementum and the periodontal membrane, which fix the teeth in the alveolar periosteum (periodontium), also originate from the mesoblastic dental sac. It is very important to systematically integrate the teeth into the cranial osteopathic test and to normalize any fixations of the teeth.

The clavicle, which comes from the membranous model, is the first bone of the embryo to begin to ossify (thirtieth day in vitro). It is also the last bone of the adult skeleton to complete its ossification (twenty-fifth year of life). This explains why we often find intraosseous lesions at this level. The clavicle is, etymologically, as well as osteopathically, an essential feature of human biomechanics. (Quadrupeds do not have clavicles.)

The organogenesis of the vertebrae is preceded by the development of mesoblastic tissue. Each of the vertebral segments originates from the sclerotome of the somites, which surrounds the dorsal chord. Once the vertebrae are ossified, the dorsal chord will progressively disappear and only the nucleus pulposus of the intervertebral disk will remain. The complete ossification of the spine is completed during the twenty-fourth year of life.

Embryologically, the ribs are an extension of the costal part of the thoracic vertebrae. The primary ossification center of a rib is precisely at the posterior rib angle. We test costotransverse and costovertebral articulation by applying pressure and/or traction at this posterior rib angle.

Certain bones, such as the sacrum and the sternum, are formed by the late fusion of the different pieces that form them. That these bones are segmental components dictates our approach toward the sacral vertebrae and the sternebrae as individual biomechanical modules. This gives much more precision to our tests, and to the efficiency of our osteopathic treatment.

In general, we should remember that the 350 bones that we have at birth will become, after the various fusions are complete, 200 bones in the adult skeleton. In their structure, bones retain the tissular imprint of the cartilaginous fusion, which previously separated its different elements. Therefore, a considerable number of intraosseous architectural and biomechanical features must be considered. For example, the bowing lesion of the tibia, which is common in the newborn, appears to be due to the constraints of the fetal position. This often leads to a valgus clubfoot deformation, which cannot be treated as a simple articular problem. The same goes for the exaggerated anteversion of the neck of the femur, which leads to a compensatory internal rotation of the hip. (The parents often consult a doctor because their child walks with one foot, or both feet, turned in.) Many orthopedic imbalances may have an intraosseous lesion as the origin. It is the osteopath's responsibility to diagnose and treat such a lesion in a growing child, as well as in the adult, who will have retained the functional sequelae of such a lesion.

The Cardiovascular System

Just like the myofascial and osseous systems, the cardiovascular system consists of connective tissue that originates from the mesoblast. The cardiovascular system is the first functional unit to be active. Activity in the heart begins on the twenty-second day of gestation, at the moment the junction between the intra- and extra-embryo vascular network has been established. The simple tubular or rudimentary heart will become the sigmoid heart during the fourth week of gestation. The sigmoid heart is divided into right and left sides. During the fifth week the heart compartmentalizes into a quadruple-cavity heart. During this same period of time, the aortic arches will develop, to later become the great arteries originating from the heart.

The entire vascular circuit (arterial, venous, and lymphatic) comes from the mesenchyme connective tissue. As leaves grow from the branch, which nourishes them with sap, the development of the sanguine tree conditions the development of all embryonic tissue that it vascularizes.

All of the elements of the blood (red blood cells, white blood cells, and platelets) originate from the mesoderm. They are produced in the bone marrow. Because of this, the intraosseous lines of force influence the production of blood cells. The spleen and the kidney, like the heart, are organs that are formed from the mesoblast. The organogenesis of the spleen follows the organogenesis of the splenic artery. The spleen is a lobular expansion of the end of the splenic artery. The absence of the spleen is extremely rare; however, the existence of many spleens along the splenic artery is relatively common.

The kidneys, as well as the genital organs, come from the intermediary mesoblast. The kidneys successively develop into pronephron

The Mechanical Link

When viewing the concept of the mechanical link anatomically, we must think of one embryologic unit-the mesenchyme or primitive connective tissue. Three interdependent systems develop from this connective tissue: the myofascial system, the osseous system, and the cardiovascular system.

These three anatomical systems are organized into eight functional units:
1. The Spine.
2. The Thorax.
3. The Extremities.
4. The Intraosseous Lines of Force.
5. The Viscera.
6. The Cardiovascular Apparatus.
7. The Osseous Head.
8. The Derma.

All manual therapeutic approaches that are truly global should evaluate each of these functional units with equal attention because they are all equal parts of the general organization of our connective structure. Also, each unit can be the site of osteopathic lesions.

The common embryological origin of these eight functional units, in itself, justifies the concept of the osteopathic mechanical link. This concept incorporates three principle elements:
1. the connection of these different structures (the link);
2. certain similar physical properties (mechanical similarity);
3. the same manual and therapeutic action at every level (osteopathic examination and treatment).

CHAPTER 2

Anatomy of the Fasciae

Visualize a spider web that is spun in three dimensions. Like that spider web, the fasciae form a vast multidirectional network. This is due to the various orientations of the fibers. We find fasciae everywhere in the body. We can divide fasciae into many systems, at the same time remembering that the fasciae are continuous.

The first system is formed by the superficial aponeurosis. The second is formed by the cervico-thoraco-abdomino-pelvic system, which is the deep fascia. The third is the dura mater system. Also, there exists a fourth system that lines the superficial fascia and is called the superficialis fascia. All four systems of fasciae are closely linked to each other and function synergistically. If you put one under tension, it automatically transmits tension to the other levels. Therefore, an osteopathic lesion never remains isolated. It causes lesions at a distance. This global view of the fasciae allows us to understand the fundamental notion of the *total lesion*.

This mechanical link that connects different osteopathic lesions to each other includes:
- the *muscular link* that relates to the superficial fascia;
- the *vascular link* that relates to the deep fascia;
- the *neurological link* that relates to the dura mater fascia.

Because our therapeutic method is based on the anatomical reality of these lesional chains, we have named it, the *osteopathic mechanical link*.

The Superficial Fasciae

Superficial fasciae forms the external envelope of the body. The internal muscular partitions and anaponeurotic system originate from the internal surface of the superficial fasciae. The muscles are separated into functional groups, as well as into individual muscles by these internal muscular partitions and the aponeurotic system.

These muscular loggia are formed by the expansion of the superficial aponeurosis, thereby creating a strong relationship with the external environment. The superficial aponeurosis is the musculoskeletal fascia. Therefore, it is a key component for motor coordination. The superficial aponeurosis inserts around the cranium, the spine, the shoulder and pelvic girdle, as well as on certain bones of the extremities.

The degree of muscular tension is largely dependent on the state of the fascial tension. Generally, a myotonic lesion is secondary to an osteopathic fixation, and not the other way around.

We call the *anterior fasciae*, the fasciae that are situated anterior to the central line of gravity. Conversely, *posterior fasciae* are situated posterior to the central line of gravity.

Fasciae at the Level of the Head and Neck

The superficial aponeurosis is stretched between the contours of the cranium and the shoulder girdle. This superficial system is related to the inferior floor of the cranium. We can divide the superficial aponeurosis into two parts, the anterior part and the posterior part.

The Anterior Part

The anterior temporal aponeurosis inserts superiorly on the temporal line to include the parietal, the frontal, the superior border of the zygomatic arch, the posterior border of the zygoma, and the lateral crest of the frontal.

The masseter aponeurosis inserts on the superior border of the zygomatic arch, the coronoid apophysis, and on the posterior and inferior border of the mandible.

The anterior superficial cervical aponeurosis inserts superiorly onto the inferior border of the mandible, and on the masseter aponeurosis, which is a relay between the anterior superficial cervical and the temporal aponeurosis. The anterior superficial cervical aponeurosis then fixates on the anterior surface of the hyoid bone. On its inferior end it inserts

Figure 2

The Superficial Fasciae

Superficial Fasciae: Musculoskeletal Biomechanical System

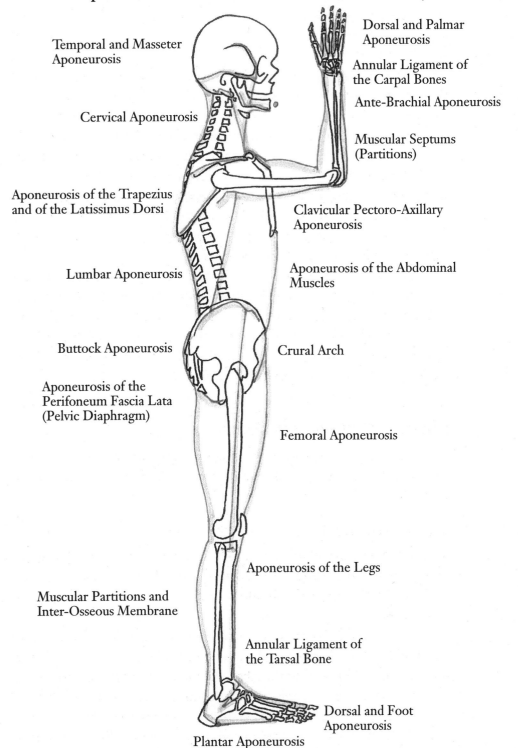

Temporal and Masseter Aponeurosis

Dorsal and Palmar Aponeurosis

Annular Ligament of the Carpal Bones

Ante-Brachial Aponeurosis

Cervical Aponeurosis

Muscular Septums (Partitions)

Aponeurosis of the Trapezius and of the Latissimus Dorsi

Clavicular Pectoro-Axillary Aponeurosis

Lumbar Aponeurosis

Aponeurosis of the Abdominal Muscles

Buttock Aponeurosis

Crural Arch

Aponeurosis of the Perifoneum Fascia Lata (Pelvic Diaphragm)

Femoral Aponeurosis

Aponeurosis of the Legs

Muscular Partitions and Inter-Osseous Membrane

Annular Ligament of the Tarsal Bone

Dorsal and Foot Aponeurosis

Plantar Aponeurosis

on the sternal notch, the anterior surface of the manubrium, and the superior surface of the clavicle.

The hyoid bone is "taken hostage" between the osseous head and the shoulder girdle. Therefore, lesions of the hyoid bone are frequent but most often an adaptation.

The Posterior Part

The posterior temporal aponeurosis inserts superiorly on the temporal line, which includes the parietal, the mastoid crest, and the external auditory canal.

The posterior superficial cervical aponeurosis inserts superiorly on the curved line of the occiput, the mastoid, and the external auditory canal. Then it inserts on the posterior part of the external surface of the hyoid bone, and descends to insert on the scapular spine and then on the acromion. On its internal surface—a sagittal expansion—the posterior cervical ligament attaches it to the spinous process of the cervical vertebrae and the first four thoracic vertebrae.

At the level of the shoulder girdle, the posterior superficial cervical aponeurosis has common insertions with those of the trunk and the upper extremities. This causes the shoulder girdle to be a very important relay of fascial tension. And except for direct trauma at this level, the cervical vertebrae are essentially a compensatory zone. Therefore, before adjusting a cervical lesion, the cause must be found.

Fasciae at the Level of the Trunk

The superficial aponeurosis is stretched from the shoulder girdle to the pelvic girdle. It is comprised of the anterolateral part and the posterior part.

The Anterolateral Part

The clavi-pectoro-axillary aponeurosis and the aponeurosis of the pectoralis major and the serratus muscle form the thoracic fascia. This fascia links the thorax to the shoulder girdle, and thereby, to the upper extremities.

The abdominal fascia is formed by the aponeurosis of the abdominal obliques. The insertion of the abdominal obliques is mixed with the thoracic unit at the level of the ribs. The multidirectional pattern of the oblique fibers and the thoracic unit forms a crossed diagonal system between the pelvis and the shoulder girdle. This crisscross system forms a relationship between the right shoulder and the left ilium, as well as between the left shoulder and the right ilium. These fibers insert inferior on the pubic bone, the iliac crest, and the inguinal ligament. The frequency of iliac lesions in intraosseous torsion demonstrates the importance of the constraints that apply to this level.

The abdominal fascia also has longitudinal fibers that are stretched from the anteromedial part of the thorax to the pubic bone. It corresponds with the anterior rectus system. There are also transversal fibers that form the transverse aponeurosis of the abdomen. Underneath all these aponeurosis, we find the transversalis fascia. This explains all the sequelae that follow scarring in that area. Therefore it is very important to systematically test the tissular quality of abdominal scars.

At the level of the anterolateral border, we should note the importance of the inguinal ligament. It is stretched from the anterosuperior iliac spine to the pubic tubercule. In actuality, it serves as the insertion for the above-mentioned crossed system, and also for the insertion of the transversalis fascia. These various components participate in the external vascular iliac girdle. The femoral aponeurosis, the iliac fascia, and the vascular girdle of the lower extremities all insert on the inguinal ligament. The inguinal ligament is considered a crossroads between the superficial and the deep fasciae. We will systematically test it during the examination of the pelvic area.

The Posterior Part

The thoracic fascia is formed by the aponeurosis of the inferior trapezius, which is attached to the scapular spine, and the spinous process of the thoracic vertebrae. The lumbar fascia inserts on the spinous process of T–7 to S–5 vertebrae, and on the posterior quarter of the iliac crest. It gives rise to the insertion of the latissimus dorsi, which connects it to the upper extremities.

Fasciae at the Level of the Perineum

This aponeurosis system is divided into three parts that include the following:
- the superficial aponeurosis;
- the mid-aponeurosis;
- the deep or pelvic aponeurosis.

Although this division of the perineum aponeurosis is the same as that made in classical medicine, it should be made clear that the whole thing belongs to the superficial aponeurosis system. The obturator membrane also belongs to the superficial fascial system. It should be tested on its internal and external surface, as it is prone to lesions.

Fasciae at the Level of the Lower Extremities

This superficial aponeurosis is formed by the aponeurosis of the buttocks, the thigh, the lower legs, and the feet. The buttocks aponeurosis inserts on the iliac crest, the sacrum, and the coccyx. The femoral aponeurosis of the thigh is a continuation of the aponeurosis of the buttocks. Anteriorly and superiorly it is attached to the inguinal ligament. It is linked to the femur only by intermuscular separations that originate from its deep surface. Inferiorly, it is fixated to the lateral border of the patella, the patellar ligament, the tibial tuberosity, and the head of the fibula. This explains external patella lesions, external lateral lesions of the tibia, and lesions of diastasis of the superior tibiofibular articulation.

Laterally at the knee, the femoral aponeurosis gives expansion to the bicipital tendon. Medially it gives expansion to the semitendinosous and sartorius tendons. The femoral aponeurosis has a thickening on its lateral surface from the iliac crest to Gerdy's tubercule on the tibia. This thickening is called the *fasciae latae*. The fasciae latae follows the lateral intraosseous line of force of the ilium and the femur.

The aponeurosis of the leg attaches to the anterior surface of the tibia. It is linked posterior to the bones by the intramuscular separations, and then directly attaches on the malleoli and the calcaneum. The interosseous membrane, which links the tibia and fibula, must be tested during the examination of the lower leg. The aponeurosis of the lower leg is attached anterior to the annular ligaments of the tarsal bones.

The aponeurosis of the feet is divided into two parts, the dorsal and plantar. The dorsal aponeurosis covers the extensor tendons of the toes. On the side of the foot, it links to the plantar aponeurosis. At a deep level, it is connected to the pedial aponeurosis. The plantar aponeurosis is stretched from the calcaneum to the metatarsophalangeal joints.

Fasciae at the Level of the Upper Extremities

This superficial aponeurosis is formed by the axillary aponeurosis, brachial aponeurosis, antebrachial aponeurosis, and the aponeurosis of the hand.

At the level of the shoulder, the aponeurosis of the upper extremities is well connected to the aponeurosis of the trunk. This connection occurs by way of the intermediary of the aponeurosis of the pectoralis major, the axillary aponeurosis and its clavi-pectoro-axillary part, and the aponeurosis of the latissimus dorsi. From the osteopathic point of view, it is important to note that the clavi-pectoro-axillary aponeurosis is reinforced laterally by the internal coracoclavicular ligament. This explains the importance of the coracoid for diagnosis and therapy.

At the level of the arm, the superficial aponeurosis originates from the aponeurosis of the shoulder. It forms a girdle surrounding the arm and only attaches at the olecranon of the elbow. It is linked to the humerus by intermuscular separations.

At the level of the forearm, the superficial aponeurosis is fixated on the posterior border of the ulna. It attaches at the wrist on the retinaculum. If tension is present in the forearm, one should always test for tension in the interosseous membrane that links the ulna and radius.

At the level of the hand, the superficial aponeurosis on the dorsal surface starts from the extensor retinaculum and covers the extensor muscles from the first to the fifth metacarpal bones. On the palmar surface, the superficial aponeurosis is the prolongation of the palmaris longus, which inserts superiorly on the medial epicondyle. The functional unit of the palmaris longus and the palmar aponeurosis has such a strong effect that an osteopathic lesion in this area will practically always have repercussions at the level of the elbow.

At the wrist, the superficial aponeurosis passes in front of the flexor retinaculum without fixating on it and attaches longitudinal fibers to the last four fingers. These fibers form the pretendinous bands that will then fixate to the heads of the metacarpal bones at the level of the metacarpophalangeal articulation. At the level of the fingers, the superficial aponeurosis forms a digital girdle.

The Deep Fasciae

The deep system is comprised of all the deep fasciae but should not be confused with the deep layer of the superficial aponeurosis. It is connected with the viscera and the cardiovascular system. The deep fasciae inserts at the base of the cranium, the shoulder and pelvic girdles, on the spine—except between T–5 and T–11—and finally, on the lower extremities. Therefore, we see that the deep system and the superficial aponeurosis have common insertions on the bones. We can also say that the visceral unit is suspended from the cephalic (cranial) unit, and therefore, a lesion in one will have repercussions in the other.

Figure 3

The Deep Fasciae

Deep Fasciae: Viscero-Organic Biomechanical System

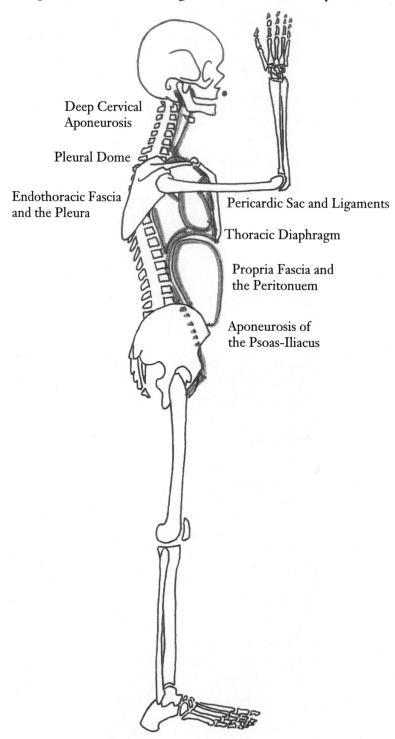

Deep Cervical
Aponeurosis

Pleural Dome

Endothoracic Fascia
and the Pleura

Pericardic Sac and Ligaments

Thoracic Diaphragm

Propria Fascia and
the Peritonuem

Aponeurosis of
the Psoas-Iliacus

Fasciae at the Level of the Head and Neck

The deep system is formed by the aponeurosis system of the pharynx, which connects the hyoid bone to the base of the cranium. It attaches to the inferior surface of the temporal and sphenoid, as well as on the pterygoid process of the sphenoid and the internal surface of the mandible. The deep system is essentially related to the middle floor of the osseous head (the maxillofacial region).

Inferior to the hyoid bone, the deep system is formed by the mid and deep cervical aponeurosis, and by the visceral girdle, which seems to be suspended from the cranium. All lesions of the viscera of the neck will have considerable effect on the biomechanics of the cranium and the cervical spine

Fasciae at the Level of the Thorax

The endopericardic fascia (or subpleural) lines the parietal sheath of the pleura. It adheres to the muscular aponeurosis and to the bones of the thorax. At the anterior surface of the spine, the deep aponeurosis continues from the cervical region to the diaphragm. However, it is strongly connected to the vertebrae until T–4.

At the pleural dome, the endopericardic fascia gives rise to a fibrous cap. This is where the suspensatory apparatus of the pleural dome inserts. The cap and the suspensatory system of the pleural dome form the fibrous cervicothoracic septum. The suspensatory apparatus of the pleural dome strongly joins the seventh cervical vertebra to the first rib. We often see fixations in this area.

Fasciae at the Level of the Mediastinum

The pleura are divided to let the pulmonary pedicle pass through it, and the pleura surrounds these pedicles. Under the hilum, its borders come together and form the ligaments of the lungs. These ligaments then descend toward the diaphragm.

The bronchodiaphragmatic membrane separates the anterior and posterior mediastinum. A reciprocal tension is created between all the organs that insert into this membrane. These organs include the bronchioles (above), the pericardium (anterior), the esophagus (posterior), the lungs (lateral) and the diaphragm (inferior). This is an area of fixation that we must examine carefully.

The pericardium is connected to the skeleton by ligaments. The vertebropericardic ligaments begin at the sagittal separations of the endopericardic fascia (deep aponeurosis) from C–7 to T–4. They are fixated on the right and left side of the superior part of this sac. The superior sternopericardic ligament, which suspends the sac from the manubrium, is fixated on the sac at the origin of the arterial trunks. The inferior sternopericardic ligament connects the inferior part of the pericardium to the inferior extremity of the sternum and to the xiphoid process. The phrenicopericardic ligaments are extensions of the endopericardic fascia.

The vascular girdles are stretched from the base of the cranium to the pericardic sac, and they are in relation with other fasciae. All osteopathic lesions of a vessel will have a biomechanical effect on neighboring osteoarticular structures.

The thoracic diaphragm represents the continuation of the deep system between the thorax and the abdomen. It is formed by a central fibrous septum in the form of a clover, the central tendon that divides it into middle, right, and left leaflets. The crura of the diaphragm border the anterior surface of the vertebrae and are lateral to the aortic opening.

The suspensatory ligament of the duodenum, the ligament of Treitz, extends to the right and left crura of the diaphragm. This connection creates a coordination of sorts between the duodenum and the diaphragm. We will systematically test the diaphragm, while remembering the ligament of Treitz.

Fasciae at the Level of the Abdomen

The deep system continues by way of the aponeurosis of the psoas muscle, which connects with the iliac fascia. In the abdomen, the deep system divides into two fascial chains that continue into the lower extremities. The aponeurosis of the psoas muscle inserts on the femur, and has a common insertion site with the iliac fascia and the femoral aponeurosis on the inguinal ligament. These common insertions demonstrate that the superficial and the deep system are continuous.

The deep abdominal system and the aponeurosis of the buttock insert on either side of the ileum. Again, we see the relation between the two systems. We can say that the superficial aponeurosis of the lower extremities is not only a part of the superficial aponeurosis system, but is also interconnected with the deep system. It is not the same for the upper extremities because the deep system does not have a direct relationship with the superficial aponeurosis in the arm. This explains why osteopathic lesions in the lower extremity will have more consequences on the total lesion than fixations in the upper extremities

Fasciae Related to the Vascular System

The vascular system mostly belongs to the deep fascial system, which connects it to all other fasciae in the body. Any fixation of an arterial segment may contribute to an osteopathic lesional chain.

Fasciae Related to the Visceral System

The thoracic and abdominal organs are connected to the deep fascial system by a play of ligaments and meso. A visceral lesion will not remain localized, but will have repercussions, by way of the deep system, on other regions of the body

The Dura Mater Fasciae

A type of fibrous tissue, the dura mater, surrounds the nervous system inside the cranium and the spine. The dura mater fascial system corresponds to the superior floor of the osseous head.

Fasciae at the Level of the Cranium

The dura mater is composed of two sheaths, which are glued together except at the venous sinuses. The external sheath lines the internal surface of the bones of the cranial vault. At the level of the sinuses, the dura mater spreads away from the bones. The internal sheath doubles over itself to form the tentorium cerebellum, the falx cerebri, and the falx cerebellum. These membranes create a reciprocal tension within the cranium. They also divide the cranial cavity, and surround the venous sinuses.

The tentorium cerebellum separates the brain from the cerebellum. The cerebral trunk passes in front of it. Its endocranial insertions are in exact relation to the exocranial insertion of the superficial fasciae. The tentorium cerebellum is the cranial diaphragm. The falx cerebri creates a sagittal (vertical) separation of the cerebral spheres. The posterior aspect of the falx cerebri is continuous laterally with the tentorium cerebellum. The falx cerebellum separates the cerebellum spheres. Similar to the falx cerebri, it has a free border anteriorly.

Figure 4

The Dura Mater Fasciae

Dura Mater Fasciae: Craniosacral Biomechanical System

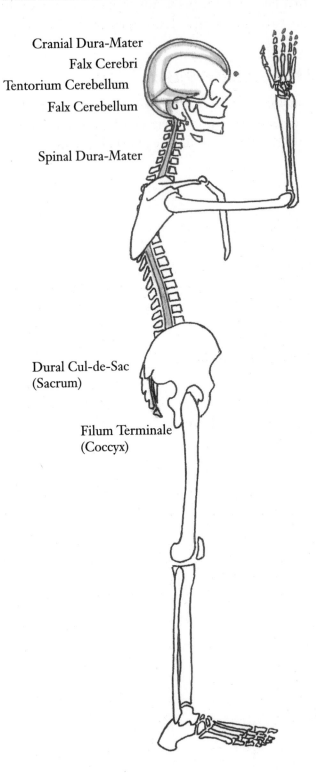

Cranial Dura-Mater
Falx Cerebri
Tentorium Cerebellum
Falx Cerebellum

Spinal Dura-Mater

Dural Cul-de-Sac
(Sacrum)

Filum Terminale
(Coccyx)

Fasciae at the Vertebral Level

The dura mater links the occiput to the sacrum and to the coccyx. Inside the vertebral canal the external sheath of the cranial dura mater is known as the *vertebral periosteum*. The spinal dura mater represents the internal sheath of the cranial dura mater. The spinal dura mater is, therefore, in direct connection with the membranes of reciprocal tension.

There are only a few osseous insertions of the spinal dura mater. They include the foramen magnum, the posterior surface of the second and third cervical vertebrae, and the anterior part of the second sacral segment. The spinal dura mater ends with the filum terminale, which goes through the sacral hiatus, and lastly, mixes with the periosteum of the coccyx.

At the level of the vertebral foramen, the dura mater branches to make room for the nerve roots. The encephalon is enveloped by the cranial dura mater, as the spinal cord is by the spinal dura mater. The peripheral nerves circulate through the fascial girdle separations (epineurium, endoneurium, and perineurium), which originate from the dura mater. Because of all this, the entire nervous system is in close relationship with the dura mater fasciae.

The Superficialis Fasciae

These fasciae play a weak role in the biomechanics of the body. However, we take them into account because they are the site of important biological action. The superficialis fasciae line the skin. They are separated from the derma by the subcutaneous tissue through which the nerves and the blood vessels travel. They cover practically all of the superficial aponeurosis throughout the body, with the exception of the face, the buttocks, the hands, and the feet.

The superficialis fasciae are closely related to all other systems of aponeurosis, especially at the level of the cranium and the inguinal ligament. This explains why a problem in one of the systems has important repercussions at the level of the superficialis fasciae functions, and vice versa.

Figure 5

The Superficialis Fasciae

Superficialis Fasciae: Biomechanical System

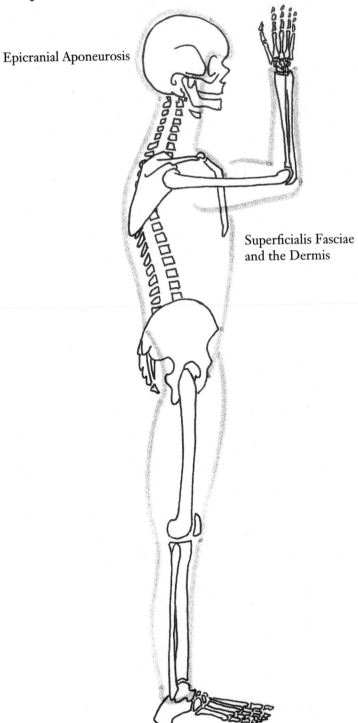

Epicranial Aponeurosis

Superficialis Fasciae
and the Dermis

3

Osteopathic Lesions

An osteopathic lesion is generally defined as being a restriction of the mobility of a structure. However, this definition is only relatively correct, and we must refine this understanding.

An osteopathic lesion is not the same as a displacement or a faulty position. The confusion between a test of mobility (dynamic) and the examination of the posture (static) is often a source of error in osteopathic diagnosis and treatment. We must make a distinction between that which *manifests* the lesion and that which *creates* the lesion. Many positional imbalances are simply an adaptation. One should never intervene on a misalignment that brings with it little or no restriction of mobility, as this may destabilize the patient. In the spirit of osteopathy and Mechanical Link, the mobility of the structure is always the critical element.

The osteopathic lesion is not so much judged by the amplitude of the movement, but by the resistance of the tissues. In fact, certain lesions, especially those related to articular diastasis, can lead to hypermobility and instability of the segment involved. The characteristic sign of an osteopathic lesion is a tissular barrier. This includes such things as a blockage, a locking, or a distinct resistance of the structure when it is put under even the smallest amount of tension.

What is the nature of this tissular resistance? The elements that determine the mechanical barrier could include articular tightness, muscular contracture, fascial tension, intraosseous rigidity, energetic cysts, or a creation of the mind. In fact, there is a histological process that clearly explains the physiological mechanism of all osteopathic lesions. This is the *scarring process of the connective tissue.*

Genesis of an Osteopathic Lesion

The scarring reaction of connective tissue that has suffered creates an osteopathic lesion. This corresponds to the expression *injured tissue*, which was first used by American osteopaths. This scarring process evolves systematically in three stages.

1. Inflammation

The inflammatory reaction is a nonspecific defense mechanism of an organism that is faced with aggression (physical trauma, chemical agent, bacterial invasion, psychological stress, etc.). Signs of inflammation include the following:

- tumor—swelling due to vasodilatation and increase of capillary permeability;
- dolor—pain due to irritation of the nervous fibers and pressure from edema;
- *calor*—heat due to local metabolic hyperactivity;
- *rubor*—redness due to an increase of vascularization and stasis of the blood.

In contractile tissues such as skeletal muscles, visceral smooth muscles, the myocardium, and the muscular covering of the arteries, this inflammatory stage is generally associated with muscle spasm. Edema and muscle spasm create excessive tension on the tissue, which constitutes the first stage of an osteopathic lesion.

Regardless of its acute, and at times, dramatic characteristics, the inflammation remains a physiological reaction that prepares for the repair of the tissue. This is normally a reversible phase. This reversal can be spontaneous or brought about with the help of a symptomatic or better global treatment.

2. Fibrosis

The fibrosis stage corresponds to a tissular reorganization that follows an inflammatory stage that was too important, too prolonged, or kept returning. The collagen fibers of the affected connective tissue increase in number and will have a different orientation depending on the constraints of the tissue. This increase of collagen fibers will create a tissular zone that is more adhesive and longer lasting. Collagen tissue sticks and is very bothersome.

The fibrosis stage of the osteopathic lesion is not spontaneously reversible. However, manual intervention that is well directed will allow a better reorganization of the tissue, and a total or partial normalization of the mobility at this level.

3. Sclerosis

This is the final stage of a pathological scarring process. Due to lack of vascularization, tissular alteration and hardening will increase. In this third stage of the osteopathic lesion we find ligamentous or tendinous calcification, exostosis, arterial sclerosis, cutaneous keratiasis, etc. Even though the sclerosis stage is not reversible (or very minimally reversible), osteopathic treatment will generally improve the adaptation capacity of the organism to this lesion. It accomplishes this by stabilizing and minimizing the tissular degradation process that has been started.

The cancerous or necrosis stage is not a true scarring process, although there is the presence of tissular suffering. The morbid predisposition of the subject's tissue evolves toward a hyperproduction of disorganized cells (cancerous) or tissular death (necrosis). Here we find the notion that is dear to homeopaths. We can now see an interesting parallel between the diathesis of an osteopathic lesion and homeopathic territory.

Figure 6

Osteopathic Diathesis and Homeopathic Territories

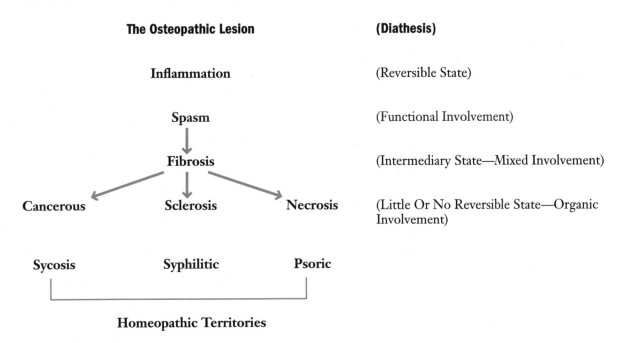

The fixation process of a tissular lesion is not always the linear process that we have described. The fibrosis stage may include inflammatory aggravation. Different stages of the lesion may coexist within the same territory. At times, even after a gentle treatment, patients report reactions such as stiffness, pain, and fatigue. This suggests that the fibrotic stage, and even the sclerotic stage, can return to the initial inflammatory stage.

To justify the necessity for a global osteopathic approach such as Mechanical Link, we must note one fundamental histological point: *connective tissue is the only cellular organization of the human body that has the ability to scar.*

This physiological characteristic of the connective tissue implies that all anatomical structures of mesodermic origin may be prone to osteopathic lesion. This includes structures such as the bones, muscles, fasciae, and blood vessels. From this point of view, muscle contracture, fascial fibrosis, articular blockage, osseous bowing, dermal fixation, visceral adhesion, or arterial spasm are all different expressions of the same lesional process. This explains why it is so important to consider all of the connective tissue as potential sites for osteopathic lesions.

At any location in the body, we can identify all osteopathic fixations with just one test. That test consists of putting the tissue under tension with manual pressure or manual traction. We can also normalize all osteopathic fixations with just one adjustment. That adjustment is the recoil (described in Chapter 6). Mechanical Link allows us to approach all cases of a lesional nature, even the most complex cases, with simplicity and coherence.

Etiology of the Osteopathic Lesion

Any factor that starts that scarring process may also be the cause of an osteopathic lesion.

Physical traumas are the most obvious possible etiology. We must include all accidents, shocks, falls, wrong movements, repetitive microtrauma, and postural lesions. We must also remember that the incident that brought the patient to the consultation is the last drop in an already-filled cup. Mechanical Link is a therapeutic choice for intervening in traumatic sequelae, from the stage of acute emergency to the most chronic condition.

Infectious pathologies also create many osteopathic lesions. Bacterial pathogens set in motion a defense mechanism and generate an inflammatory reaction. This inflammatory reaction could be the starting point for the scarring process that we have identified. If an osteopathic lesion is created, it will further create a biomechanical dysfunction, and lead to a greater vulnerability of the organism. Here we find the vicious cycle of continuous relapses. An infection creates an osteopathic lesion, which in turn facilitates a return of the illness. Mechanical Link reestablishes the normal defense mechanism of the organism. This contributes to the solution by decreasing the acute or chronic infectious pathology. Mechanical Link can be used in conjunction with other medical treatments.

Stress is a psychological factor that has a great influence on our general health. Osteopathic lesions can be created by disturbing emotions, excessive worries, intellectual overload, or any other kind of psychological distress. The stress will physically generate tensions in the body, which, if they last, will become osteopathic fixations. Mechanical Link allows us to precisely diagnosis all tissular lesions found during the examination, including somatoemotional knots. The recoil technique (mental or verbal phase, as described in Chapter 6) will help the patient to regain physical, energetic, and psychological balance.

The organism is exposed to numerous environmental disturbances caused by climate, nutrition and diet, certain medications, pollution, and the rhythm of life. These are all possible causes of osteopathic lesions. Once established, a tissular fixation may disturb the system of autoregulation and adaptation to the environment. Conversely, the neutralization of the osteopathic lesions will contribute to reinstating the homeostasis of the organism. This in turn decreases the environment's negative impact on metabolism.

The Individual Osteopathic Lesion

The individual Osteopathic lesion is the smallest identifiable osteopathic lesion found during the general examination. Examples of individual lesions include right elbow, L–5, left uterus, right vertebral artery, lateral intraosseous line of force of the left femur, tooth 23, and left C–6 dermatome. The potential number of lesions is infinite. We need a global, yet very detailed method of examination to find, if not the totality, at least the greatest number of lesions.

In Mechanical Link we have developed a systematic battery of 350 to 400 tests to quickly and completely check for the principle osteopathic fixations. Once we have identified an individual lesion, we must determine the various parameters that it encompasses. For example L–5 could be in extension, rotated left, and translated left. The specific analysis of an individual lesion will precisely define the parameters for the necessary adjustment to be done.

If a detailed analysis is applied to each segment of the body, it will show adaptive or accessory lesional parameters even on a unit where the global tests are negative. In fact, a simple restriction in flexion of L–5 will only be significant if it is strong enough to create a global lesion. That's why in the general protocol of the examination, we first apply the global tests to each individual unit. If necessary to be treated, the different parameters of the restriction can be detailed.

The Total Osteopathic Lesion

The *total osteopathic lesion* is the sum of all individual lesions that we have found during our general osteopathic examination. Each individual lesion will have a different interfering potential, and the sum of the individual lesions will greatly affect the organism. All of the individual lesions are interrelated, and the total osteopathic lesion constitutes a complex physical pathological entity. Again, we first have to look at the whole before looking at the parts in detail. The holistic vision of osteopathy must then be translated into a precise diagnosis of all the individual lesions of the patient. At the end of the treatment, we must be able to verify that all the elements of the total lesion, without exception, have regained good mobility. An osteopathic treatment must include a diagnosis of the total lesion.

The Primary Lesion

In order to normalize the numerous osteopathic lesions of a patient, it's not realistic to individually correct each one. This would only have a disturbing effect on the organism by creating an unnecessary duplication of adjustments.

Having observed this, osteopaths have come up with the concept of *primary lesion*. The primary lesion is at the center of all other lesions. By treating it, everything else will be corrected. However, this notion of the primary lesion, although rich in perspective, remains vague. To clarify this, we have to reconsider the problem based on simple and objective observations. Of all the individual osteopathic lesions that are found during the examination none have the same intensity, or the same value.

From a complete blockage to a slight restriction of mobility, there is a hierarchy of possible fixations. At the core of the total lesion, because no absolutely identical tissular tensions may coexist, one of these lesions will have a greater impact on restriction of mobility than all the others.

Our definition of the primary lesion is very concrete. It is *the individual osteopathic lesion, which during the examination of a given patient at a given moment, and in comparison with all other lesions present, has the greatest degree of tissular resistance.*

To be able to determine the primary lesion we need only to place all the lesions and restrictions that we have identified during the general examination into a hierarchy. The method and protocol of comparative evaluation to create this hierarchy can be found in the section on the inhibitory balancing test in Chapter 5. By defining the primary lesion as the major fixation of a given lesional organization, there is no confusion with the notion of the first or original lesion.

The *first* or *original lesion* is the starting point for lesional chains. It is the element that sets into motion the succession of imbalances that will take place. This is different for each person. A simple example is a sprained ankle that is the first lesion. It may lead to an ascending compensation of the ipsilateral knee, the contralateral sacroiliac joint, the fifth lumbar vertebrae, and so on. This lesional chain will be established in various ways, depending on the morphology of the person, its antecedents, other lesions that exist, and the biomechanical effect on the structure. The initial sprained ankle may not necessarily be the segment most restricted in its mobility. The primary lesion may be located at a different area of the body.

The history of the patient leads us to the symptoms (symptomatic lesion) and to the triggering event (original lesion). This will be of no help in determining the principal element of the osteopathic picture—the primary lesion. Comparing this to traditional tectonic architecture, we can consider the primary lesion to be the keystone of the osteopathic building. The original lesion is only a foundation stone of the building.

The total lesion and the primary lesion do not remain immovable entities. The lesional organization of a person is partially dependent on the time and the circumstances. For instance, the restriction of mobility of the thoracic vertebra will change in intensity after an exercise program. The fixation of the uterus will change depending on the menstrual cycle. The stomach will change in function based on the digestive phase. The total lesion remains, but it also adapts, accommodates, and acclimatizes.

That's why it is very important to understand that the primary lesion is always the one found during the examination. The primary lesion will be determined and effectively treated in the "here and now" of the examination. Therefore, it is not reasonable to establish a treatment plan based on the diagnosis of the preceding visits. The total lesion of a patient must be considered as a unique space-time element. Even after treating and seeing tens of thousands of cases, an osteopath will never do two exactly identical treatments.

CHAPTER 4

Posture and Postural Expression

The Posture

Posture is the objective study of the position of the body in space. Because all disharmony in the maintenance of the body is expressed by abnormal fascial tension, the posture will give us an image of the way the total lesion of the patient is being manifested. However—and this is an essential point that we will return to—postural examination of the subjects is of no help whatsoever to diagnose the primary lesion. In this work, checking the posture is mostly for reference, allowing us to appreciate the presence of fascial tension and to verify the results of our treatment.

We must differentiate between postural imbalance that is reversible and that which is due to the irreversible deformation of the skeleton. Thus, some hyperkyphosis or scoliosis may indicate a very disturbing static condition, whereas in another situation, it might not be a sign of serious imbalance. In any case, a Mechanical Link treatment must allow the patient to return to a harmonious and comfortable posture.

Postural Expression

Posture, for someone who can interpret it, is a physical and psychological expression of a person's character and being; thus, we use the term *postural expression*. In order to understand a subject's postural expression, we bring as evidence the notion of *diathesis*—i.e. all habitual physical and psychological behaviors to which the subject is predisposed to by nature.

To read the postural expression is not to judge the person but to better understand how she functions. Usually, the postural expression is complex because it's the reflection of many imbalances.

Visual Examination

At the beginning and at the end of each visit, we observe the patient standing up in a natural position, with the legs slightly apart, the arms hanging along the sides of the body, looking straight in front. We describe the posterior view and the side view.

Posterior View Inspection

From the back, postural imbalances are revealed by a disharmony of the vertebral axis. A vertebral deviation could take different forms: a right

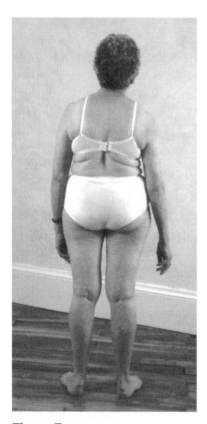

Figure 7

Simple Posterior View: Thoracic Side-Bending Right

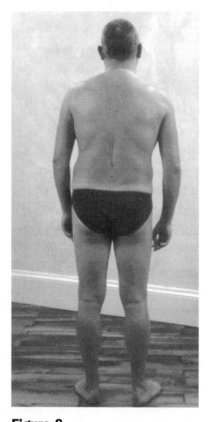

Figure 8

Complex Posterior View: Left Lateral Translation of the Pelvis and Thoracic Right Side-Bending

or left lateral inclination (superficial fascial tension); a right or left lateral translation (deep fascial tension). The lateral translation is characterized by a rupture of the line between the spinous process; it corresponds to a more established stage of the total lesion.

Depending on which vertebral level is implicated, the postural dystonia will not have the same significance:

- The superior level (cephalic) is related to the mental.
- The middle level (thoracic) is related to the rhythmic functions, such as respiration, those of the cardiovascular system, and the emotions.
- The inferior level (abdominopelvic) is related to all basic functions of organisms such as digestion, sexuality, or the need for security.

Side View Inspection

Interpretation of postural expression must also take into account the observation of the side view. From the side, we essentially look at the posture in relation to the line of gravity, at the three vertebral levels. In cases of marked fascial tension, we can expect visible compression disorganization. Imbalance can occur in more than one level in anterior or posterior flexion: in superficial fascial tension or in translation (deep fascial tension). An anterior imbalance corresponds to a hyperfunction and to excessive activity turned towards the outside; a posterior imbalance is a hypofunction and a much more reserved behavior.

Evaluation

An imbalance will be interpreted depending on which level is implicated, but being very careful to take into account the vertebral alignment itself. Therefore, an anterior rolling of the shoulder—a frequent posture seen in young girls around puberty—is often a posterior displacement of the thoracic level, in other words, a reserved behavior and not an extroverted behavior.

In addition to these anterior and posterior imbalances, we must talk about one more, the *compression* posture, where the patient seems to have lost her normal height: as if she has the weight of the world on her shoulders. This compression results from a deep fascial tension and/ or dura mater tension. It is translated into a lack of energy, established fatigue: and the patient feels as if he or she has no "bounce." With a bit of sharpness during the observation, we can notice if this compression is global or at a particular vertebral level.

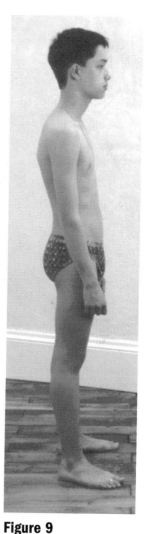

Figure 9

Side View: Global Compression and Anterior Translation of the Head

During the evaluation stage of each visit we make a diagram of the postural imbalance of each patient. We can describe the intensity of each imbalance, assigning a numerical value that indicates the severity.

After the treatment, it's interesting to observe our subject again. If the posture has normalized, our prognostic will be a favorable resolution of the problem. On the contrary, if it has remained unchanged, the improvement will be minimal and will not last long.

Visual examination of the posture is especially useful when working with children with scoliosis because the posture is still reversible, depending on the functional stage of vertebral deformation. If we can obtain a satisfactory postural balance, we can then neutralize the evolution process of the scoliosis. The systematic observation of the postural behavior also allows the parents to appreciate the results of our treatments.

The posture is also an interesting reference for judging the effects of orthotics. If after an osteopathic treatment, a patient wonders if he or she should still wear the orthotics, we only have to observe the person with the orthotics and shoes and then with bare feet. If the orthotics worsen the postural behavior, we should not hesitate to advise him or her to stop wearing them. If wearing the orthotics improves the posture, the patient should be advised to continue wearing them. If wearing the orthotics doesn't change anything, the patient may decide whether to wear them or not.

In general, the systematic observation of the postural expression is an objective method:

- to evaluate the organization and the importance of the lesional pattern;
- to verify the results of our treatment;
- to follow the evolution of the patient in time.

However, comprehensive diagnosis of the presence of osteopathic lesions surely remains in the domain of palpatory examination, and this is covered in the following chapter. Visual inspection is only the beginning.

CHAPTER 5

The Tests

The Determination of an Osteopathic Lesion

We have seen in an earlier chapter that we can consider an osteopathic lesion as being a restriction of mobility in a particular body structure. This fixation is characterized by an abnormal resistance in the connective tissue of this structure.

With this understanding we can now approach the practical method of how to manually diagnose the tissular lesion—an essential question because the osteopathic treatment depends on this point. How can we determine the osteopathic legion with a precise, objective, and reliable method?

With Mechanical Link, we simply apply only one test: we put a particular body segment under tissular tension, meaning to manually provoke fascial tension in the examined structure. How we induce the tension varies: we may do it through pressure, by traction, or by combining the two.

As a result of this test, we will experience under our hands one of two possible responses: softness and elasticity of the tissue, indicating a free structure (negative test); or a clear and marked resistance of the tissue, indicating an osteopathic lesion (positive test). As surprising as it may be, we use only this type of test because it has considerable advantages.

- It is an easy test because we only have to push or pull gently on a particular body element.
- It is practical at all levels (vertebral, thoracic, extremities, visceral, vascular, etc.). All functional units, without exception, can be examined this way.
- We can use this test with all patients, no matter what age (babies and children, adults, the elderly), what type of constitution or state of health.
- It is a very easy test for the practitioner as well as for the patient because we do not need any particular positioning, no difficult mobilization and even in very painful cases we keep the tissue tension below the pain threshold. In general, the movement is soft, using ten, twenty, thirty grams of pressure, which correctly applied, is enough to find a positive blockage if it exists.
- It is an objective, reliable, and precise test, as much in its execution as in the response. Different practitioners will find the same results for the same test, and the patient also may feel the difference between a positive or negative test.
- It is an extremely rapid test that gives an instant response; this rapidity of application allows us to make 350 to 400 tests during our normal consultation.
- It is a simple test, and results are reproducible, so it is very useful for verifying the corrections that have been made.

Examination Protocol

We have to agree with the late Thomas Dummer, D.O. when he affirmed in his seminars that osteopathy is seventy-five percent examination and twenty percent treatment. To totally decipher the lesional organization of a patient requires a methodical palpatory examination that includes several elements:

- *global tests* of each biomechanical segment that is susceptible to lesion;
- *inhibitory balancing tests* which allow us to compare and place in hierarchy the different fixations found;
- *specific tests* to analyze in detail each individual lesion that must be treated;
- *verification tests* to control the efficiency of our adjustment.

The Global Tests

The global tests work by putting individual biomechanical segments under tension, and are an indispensable shortcut that allows us to find out if there is a significant lesion in particular areas.

To optimally cover all functional units we need about 350 systematic global tests. Such a complete and necessary diagnostic procedure is only possible if we can rapidly follow a very organized series of tests. With experience we have developed a sequence of tests, carrying out global tests within each functional unit, in roughly this order:

- OVP (occipito-vertebral-pelvic) axis and the posterior thorax;
- anterior thorax;
- extremities;
- intraosseous lines of force;
- viscera and organs;
- vascular system;
- cranium;
- skin.

Once we have completed these global tests we will be able to clearly identify the exact number and the precise location of all individual lesions that make up the total lesion. All the individual osteopathic lesions that we have found will be written down on specially designed charts. We usually find between ten and thirty individual lesions in a patient who has been correctly examined from head to toe.

However, it must be noted that while global tests will tell us with certainty if there are individual osteopathic lesions, these tests do not give us any information on the restrictive parameters that have caused them. For example, the global tests of a vertebral segment might determine a global fixation of L–1 but will not reveal if the lesion is in flexion, extension, side-bending, rotation, compression, or lateral translation, or if it is an intraosseous lesion. That's why treatment of an individual lesion depends on the use of specific tests that we will explain later on.

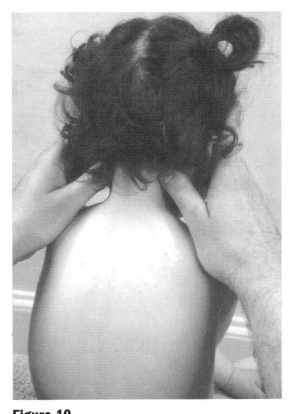

Figure 10
Global Test of the Occiput

The Inhibitory Balancing Test

This takes us to the heart of the Mechanical Link method: the balancing system that represents a modus operandi for discovering the primary lesion.

- With the observation of the posture, the total lesion is visible.
- With the global test, the total lesion is readable.
- With the inhibitory balancing test, the total lesion becomes intelligible.

The balancing system allows us to decipher the lesional pattern of the patient. Once we have identified all the lesions present in our subject, we then need to be able to establish a hierarchy that shows their relationship to one another. To do so, we will use *the inhibitory balancing test*, a comparative test that allows us to logically and rigorously find, with a high degree of certainty, the dominant lesions of the patient. The inhibitory balancing test compares the osteopathic lesions to one another in order to determine which one has the most tension.

In practice, this test is supported by a simple observation. When you place your hands on two different fixations (a simultaneous tension test), a curious phenomenon immediately happens: one of the two lesions lets go, while the other one persists. Obviously, the fixation that persists will be considered dominant in relation to the one that has been neutralized.

Figure 11

Inhibitory Balance Test of the Liver and of the Right Frontal Sinus

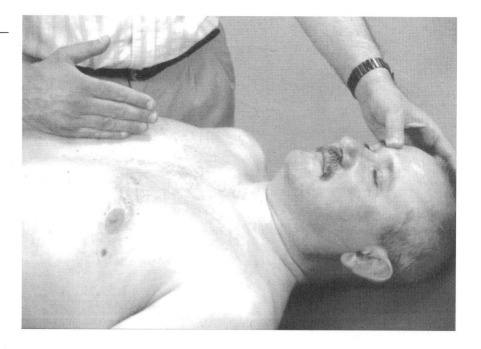

Under our hands we have the sensation that one of the fascial tensions is being reinforced while the other one is disappearing, as if the secondary lesion were being deactivated.

The physiological mechanism that explains the inhibitory reflex needs to be scientifically studied; however, without any doubt it must be due to a neurological phenomenon that puts into play the mechanoreceptors of the connective tissue. In any case, we have made use of this phenomenon for almost twenty-five years with consistent results. The testimony of numerous manual therapists trained in Mechanical Link also confirms the astounding reliability of the inhibitory balancing test.

The inhibitory balancing test is effective for comparing all existing osteopathic lesions. We can confront a point of tension in the viscera with a vertebral blockage, a costal fixation with a place of cutaneous scarring, an intraosseous lesion with an arterial spasm, and so on.

For obvious reasons of organization and convenience, we do not perform these tests at random but within each functional unit as we examine it. For example, if with the global tests we have found several vertebral restrictions, we must compare them to find out which is more severe. For this, we will compare the two extreme vertebrae (the highest and the lowest ones) by applying simultaneous pressure on the spinous process near both of them. The vertebra that resists will be compared to the next vertebra. We will proceed by successive elimination and, by always keeping the vertebral segment that resists the most, we will have the final result: the dominant lesion of the spine (the one that represents the most severe restriction of mobility.)

Using the same protocol, we then define the major fixation (dominant lesion) in each of these other seven functional units, which will give us a total picture:
- the occipito-vertebro-pelvic axis and the posterior thorax;
- the anterior thorax;
- the upper and lower extremities;
- the intraosseous line of force;
- the viscera;
- the cardiovascular system;
- the osseous head;
- the derma.

We will obtain, at the most, eight dominant lesions, because some functional units may be clear of lesion.

At the final stage of the examination, we only need to do the inhibitory balancing test between the dominant lesions, using this simple and accurate method of successive elimination of the less restricted lesion. The most resistant lesion of all, the dominant of the dominant lesions, is called the *primary lesion*.

The Specific Tests

Once global tests have determined fixations, and inhibitory balancing tests have determined which is the primary lesion, there is one last step to the examination. Even when we know which is the primary or dominant lesion, we still have to find the parameters of fixation. *The specific test* will be used to analyze all the possible restrictions of mobility in individual osteopathic lesions that need to be treated.

The tests consist of putting a selected body segment under tension in all degrees of possible minor movements. For example if we need to analyze the dominant lesion of the knee, we need to analyze all its biomechanical movements by the following specific tests:

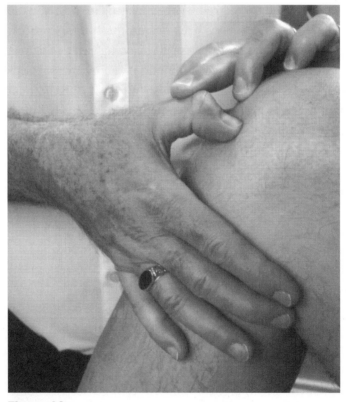

Figure 12

Specific Test: Anterior Horn of the Medial Meniscus of the Right Knee

- anterior and posterior drawer test of the tibia;
- internal and external rotation of the tibia;
- internal and external translation of the tibia;
- abduction (valgus), adduction (varus) of the tibia;
- internal and external lateral rolling of the femoral condyle;
- decompression (traction) of the femoral condyle in relation to the tibia;
- lowering and elevation of the patella;
- lateral and medial displacement of the patella;
- clockwise and counterclockwise rotation of the patella;
- anterior and posterior lowering and elevation of the fibular head;
- lateral distraction of the fibular head;
- movement of the anterior and posterior horn of the internal and external meniscus.

We don't mention the articular diastasis lesion of the fibulotibial articulation or the intraosseous lesion of the knee because they will be investigated later, in the general examination of the lines of force.

Once we have done this battery of tests, if there are many parameters in lesion, we now have to do the inhibitory balance test of the different degrees of restriction to find the dominant parameter.

With the articulation of the knee, once we have done the specific tests we may have found an anterior tibia lesion, and ones related to the external patella and the posterior horn of the internal meniscus. The balance tests will allow us to order (in hierarchy) these three fixations, to find the major restriction of the knee. The necessity of the specific test should now be clear: to normalize the knee in its entirety we have to act where it is most necessary, i.e. upon the dominant blockage of this lesion. The precision of the diagnostic, and its detail, makes for the treatment's efficiency.

Tests and More Tests

After carrying out the global tests, the inhibitory balancing tests, and the specific tests, we will be able to identify the primary osteopathic lesion and its specific degree of dominant restriction. The adjustment by recoil that we practice will be applied directly to this last parameter, in order to liberate the maximal point of tension that locks this lesion. And, after the correction, again we must use our tests! It is necessary to verify the efficiency of our treatment because we want to influence all lesions that we have noted. We verify the efficacy of the treatment by simply repeating the previously positive global tests of the general examination.

Most important is to make sure that the primary lesion has been normalized by the adjustment of its major parameter. If that is not the case, we will now retest all degrees of restriction of the specific parameters to find the one that has resisted. After the adjustment of the second most dominant parameter, we check—always by means of the global tests—the normality of the lesion in its entirety.

Once the primary lesion has been released, we then have to make sure that the secondary lesions have also been neutralized. We reexamine all individual lesions that we have noted in the general examination. Usually a great number of the lesions will have also been normalized by the simple adjustment of the primary lesion. That is the beauty of having created a hierarchy and of being able to address the primary lesion first.

If certain fixations remain, again they must be balanced against one another to determine the most dominant one. This dominant lesion, just as with the primary lesion, will be analyzed by doing specific tests relevant to the area to be treated, in order to find the major restriction upon which we will perform the next adjustment.

To review, after finishing the general examination and finding the primary lesion and its dominant specific parameter to be treated, we perform the recoil. Then we retest to determine that the specific lesion has released, and also retest to make sure the global lesion has released. We then retest all individual lesions previously found to verify the efficacy of our recoil. After that we perform the inhibitory balancing test to find the second dominant lesion—and repeat the procedure.

We continue in this way until we achieve neutralization of the total lesion, i.e. until all the individual lesions that we had diagnosed during our general examination have been neutralized. It may seem as though this method requires too much testing! However, though they are all indispensable, their rapidity of execution allows them to be used as necessary without adding too much time to consultations. In any case, the time spent doing testing is always time gained because an exact diagnostic will make possible a very efficient treatment.

CHAPTER 6

The Recoil

Choice of Technique

If palpatory diagnostics answers the problem of *where to act*, choice of treatment asks the question of *how to act*.

The therapeutic repertoire of osteopaths normally allows them to adapt to all situations because in their "toolbox" they have a vast number of techniques, known as direct, semi-direct, indirect, functional, myotensive, reflexive, neuromuscular, pumping, articular mobilization, etc. However, we have noticed that the profusion and variety of techniques do not necessarily improve the quality of care.

Has the evolution of different manual approaches brought us farther away from the simple and efficient gestures developed by Still? Before we present our recoil technique, it is useful to review how the founder of osteopathy himself practiced, the features of his work:

- Simple techniques. Still used the same principles of tissular stretching and articular mobilization to treat all regions of the body.
- Direct techniques. The "good old doctor" always tried to directly correct the lesions, by applying a force that was opposite to the resistance.
- Techniques without "thrust." Still worked on different tissular restriction that fixated the osteopathic lesion, without any manipulation (thrust).
- Rapid techniques. Corrections were made in a very short adjustment periods, at the most of a few minutes' duration. This limited excessive

intervention once the tissues were released. ("Find it; fix it; leave it.")

- Comfortable techniques. As much out of respect for the patient as in the interest of efficiency, the methods of Still were never dangerous, aggressive, or painful.

Even if the choice of treatment rests upon sound reasoning, personal conviction, and professional competence all therapeutic acts imply complete responsibility on the part of the one who performs them. We sincerely believe that Still's technical criteria should remain a common reference for all osteopaths.

Principles and Advantages of the Recoil

We know that the osteopathic lesion is characterized by a tissular fixation that manual treatment will liberate in the most physiological way possible. For us, no matter which body structure is involved, we propose the same gesture: *the recoil*.

Inspired a little by the *toggle recoil* of chiropractors, but considerably decreasing the corrective force of the manipulation, over time we developed an original technique specific to Mechanical Link. Although the adjustment that we practice nowadays has little to do with the chiropractic maneuver, we have, however, retained the term *recoil* with reference to the visible rebound of the hand once the movement is finished. In Mechanical Link the recoil is much lighter, much less intense; the direction is very precise and three-dimensional; it is very quick, and the hands are removed in order to let the vibration go through. There is only one point of contact. The correction is done by breaking the barrier (implosion) whereas in the toggle recoil it is through release that the correction is made. The Mechanical Link recoil works on the mechanoreceptors that react to position, direction, speed, and vibration. The Mechanical Link recoil is always done by direct correction, by pushing against the barrier.

The technique consists of liberating the fixation by applying, against the resistance of the tissue, a very sharp and subtle impulse. Before describing the gesture involved, we first would like to explain the numerous advantages of the recoil.

The recoil is an efficient technique, one of the most efficient and powerful of all in the osteopathic arsenal. The position of impact makes the adjustment possible no matter what type of lesion, how severe the tension, or how long it has been present. With the recoil the osteopathic treatment gains softness, depth, and sheer ability of action because the efficiency of good tissular normalization depends most of all on the quality of the gestures.

The recoil is a simple and logical technique, because it's a natural extension of the test that revealed the lesion. The recoil does not necessitate any particular positioning of the patient, acrobatic contortion of the osteopath, drop table, or other such sophisticated material. It is a relatively easy technique that students can practice immediately with quite good results. And while perfection of a maneuver may only be obtained through daily repetition, since the same movements are always used, mastery of the technique is rapid. The recoil can be easily adapted to many different situations, for treating all articular fixations—visceral, intraosseous, and arterial—all possible imaginable osteopathic lesions.

The recoil is a structural technique, in other words a direct technique, because the impulse of the movement is always directed against the resistance of the tissues that are in lesion. The rebound characteristic of the adjustment is only the quick release of the hand once the corrective gesture is finished. With the recoil we don't want to rebound against the structure but only to remove the hand as soon as the adjustment has been done so that we do not interfere with the vibrational impact that has been transmitted to the tissues.

The recoil is a nonmanipulative technique because there is no thrust, not even mobilization of the structure to be treated. We create tension by applying a few grams of pressure or by applying traction, and the corrective push does not create any displacement. Why push, right up to structural limits, if applying minimum pressure is sufficient and well below the pressure applied by the usual manipulation? Do we really need a cracking to justify an articular correction? The possible contraindications, inconvenience, and limitations of manipulation, even well executed, are numerous, and the apprehension of patients can also be understood. We don't want to give the impression that we are criticizing the traditional osteopathic articular manipulation that we ourselves have practiced for many years with some results. However, with all respect, we must claim that the recoil represents clear progress toward the security and efficiency of therapeutic gestures.

The recoil is an extremely rapid adjustment technique and only needs a few seconds to apply. With Mechanical Link, the efficacy of the treatment is always surprising because it takes so little time and brings immediate results, not just release of the lesion that is the focus, but also numerous secondary fixations that depend on it. Therefore, just one recoil can simultaneously liberate many osteopathic lesions situated in various parts of the body. Even if the efficacy of the therapeutic act is not measured by the speed of its execution, a short treatment allows us not to intervene too much, and leaves a lot more time for the examination and diagnostic procedures.

The recoil is a very comfortable, inoffensive, and painless technique. The recoil can be applied to sensitive or fragile structures: osteoporosis, fractures, the site of surgeries, with or without surgical hardware, and to places of very acute suffering, even a severe herniated disk, and so on.

With almost any therapeutic approach there are some occasions that it is not indicated because we only treat the functional part of a problem, and other medical treatments may be more indicated for severe organic pathologies. But, even in these cases, the treatment by recoil will not do damage and often allows release and improvement for patients. The physician's dictum to *do no harm* must remain a golden rule for the osteopath. The choice of the recoil, with the perfect security that it offers, authorizes us to approach without hesitation delicate problems with which we are regularly confronted.

The recoil is a technique that has evolved over the years. Actually, we propose many possible variations of the recoil, from the basic technique to the very latest stages that have potential and that are still in the research stage. We will describe here the first four phases of the recoil that we use the most often in our regular practice, and we will talk a little bit about the other, more experimental phases that are reserved for use of advanced practitioners.

The Recoil—Phase One

The basic version of the recoil has been used for many years, and we teach it to beginners in Mechanical Link. It is used in all cases. The recoil is practiced in the same position as the tension test. The first part of the maneuver is to use pressure or traction to find the point of blockage of the osteopathic lesion. For example, for a vertebra in flexion lesion, we must put the pad of the thumb on the superior border of the spinous process, and gently extend the vertebral segment until we meet the fascial resistance that maintains the blockage in flexion (motor barrier).

For the second part of the recoil, we need to go beyond the tissular barrier by giving a very short and very rapid impulse against the resistance. The impact of the recoil must be seen as a *microsurgical hit* which will *explode* the fixation that causes the problem and produce shock waves that will have a repercussion on the whole implicated lesional chain. In this case, the vibration that is being produced by the recoil will not only instantaneously reduce the lesion upon which we have applied the technique but will also act at a distance upon the secondary fixations that depends on it in the hierarchy of the lesions.

This simple adjustment and the chain reaction that it provokes can liberate a great number of lesions at once. This distant correction will naturally be verifiable; testing will show immediate normalization of tissues that previously tested positive during the examination. However, it should be noted that this economy of treatment is obviously only possible if the recoil has been judiciously applied to a primary or dominant lesion. If the technique is done on a secondary restriction, or during the symptomatic targeting treatment, the efficiency of the recoil will remain local.

Figure 13

The Recoil

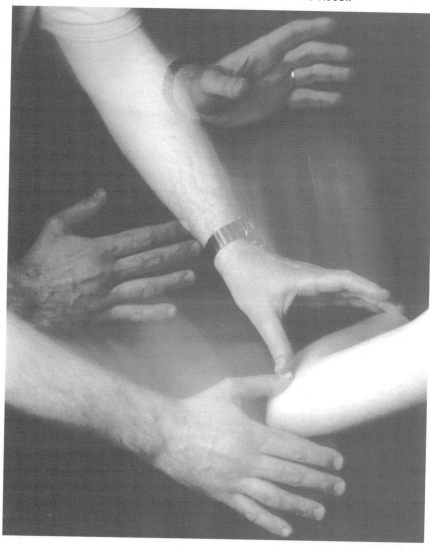

The purpose of phase one of the recoil is to directly unblock an osteopathic lesion at the site of its restriction, i.e. in the major parameter of the lesion. If the recoil is not enough to completely liberate the fixation, it can be repeated many times in the same direction or on other parameters of the lesion until normalization occurs. Compared with classical manipulation technique, the recoil has the advantage of being able to be repeated as necessary, and beginners need not be fearful if they have to apply the technique many times to get good results!

The Recoil—Phase Two

The second phase of the recoil makes use of the same movement as that used in phase one but adds precision to the tension it puts on the lesion. By varying the orientation of the finger—held in the same position as it is in phase one—we do a vertical sweep from the fascial barrier that we have already found, then a horizontal one, and then a rotation one. In this way we define, in all three dimensions, the principal location of the lesion. This three-dimensional sweep allows us to concentrate our action on the precise point of the tissular fixation to treat, considerably increasing the efficiency as well as the reach of the recoil. This is a *three-dimensional* adjustment of the lesion!

The Recoil—Phase Three

At some point, many years ago, when we were practicing the recoil up to phase two only, we had the idea to observe the possible variations of an osteopathic lesion with reference to the subject's breathing. Asking the patient to breathe slightly more deeply than usual allowed us to observe that during a certain part of the inhalation or exhalation, the fixation is clearly increased. This increase of the fascial resistance during one of the two breathing phases is always independent of the mechanical movement, or thoracic amplitude. Thus, in different subjects the same blockage in flexion of the vertebra might increase during inhalation while for others it might be during exhalation. The articular physiology that automatically associates the extension of the spine with inhalation, and inversely, flexion with thoracic exhalation, has no influence on the intensity of the concerned tissular restriction.

In respiration, inhalation naturally corresponds to an anabolic phase (assimilation and synthesis), whereas, exhalation relates to the catabolic phase (dissipation and elimination). The parasympathetic part of the autonomic nervous system is in charge of the anabolic process, while the sympathetic part stimulates the catabolic reactions of the organism. In the dialect of Chinese energy medicine, the anabolic phase corresponds to the *yin* phase and the catabolic with its opposed and complimentary *yang* phase.

Psychologically, the inhalation relates to a mental or emotional feeling of refreshing and recharging, whereas the exhalation corresponds to a process of letting go and abandonment. In general, and no matter which level of blockage—physical, metabolic, or psychological—as long as the recoil is done at the moment of maximum tension, no matter at which particular point of the respiration this may be, it will have a powerful and wide-ranging effect.

In classical articular manipulation, we use the relaxation phase of the muscle that accompanies the exhalation to thrust. However, even if the intention behind this seems good, it will impose on the structure an exhalation phase that may not correspond to the necessity of the organism. The solution to adapt to each case seems to be simple and physiologically logical because one only needs to notice if the lesion is increased with inhalation or exhalation and then make the adjustment during the respiration phase that corresponds to the increase of tissular restriction.

In practice, after putting the fascial barrier under tension following the parameters of phases one and two, the patient is asked to inhale slowly and deeply and then to exhale the same way. On the first respiration cycle, the practitioner observes at which moment of the inhalation or exhalation the blockage increases (the tension of the fascial barrier will increase under the finger) and during the next respiration cycle, the recoil is done at the point of increased tension.

With this third phase, the corrective movement of the recoil not only becomes more efficient at increasing biomechanical normalization of the lesion, but also at reaching the secondary fixations at a distance.

The Recoil—Phase Four

The fourth phase of the recoil arises from the outcome of work in the preceding phase. Once it is clear whether restriction is increased upon inhalation or exhalation, the patient is asked to stop breathing at the precise moment of increased tension. The inhalation or exhalation apnea will then lock in even more strongly the fixation to be treated, as well as all fascial chains that are connected to it. At that point, it will seem that the lesional pattern has been maximized in its totality, and the impact of the recoil will cover considerably more territory than it did with the preceding phases.

The fourth phase of the recoil—due to its great intensity and range of covering secondary lesions—is the one that we generally use for treating primary and dominant fixations.

The Experimental Phases of the Recoil

There are still more phases of the recoil, corresponding to more subtle levels of treatment, and these constitute one direction of research and evolution in our practice of Mechanical Link. At these levels the principle of the recoil remains the same, but by introducing new parameters we try to increase the fascial tension of the osteopathic lesion, and to orient our action in a particular therapeutic direction.

The Phase of Tissular Respiration

Repeating a protocol similar to that of phase four, the phase we call *tissular respiration* is based on movements other than pulmonary respiration. It is known that our bodies are moved by numerous rhythms: that of thoracic respiration, the primary respiratory mechanism of the cerebrospinal fluid, the heartbeat, that gives arterial pulse, the lymphatic fluctuations, the proper motility of the viscera, etc. Our organism doesn't just play one musical instrument: it plays a great symphony—the symphony of life. We call *global respiratory movement* the sum of all different perceptible biorhythms felt by our hands, rhythms that we will use to do the recoil.

The first step is to start from the parameters of phase two and listen to the blockage. After a few seconds of floating, the general respiratory movement—or more exactly the progressive increase of the tissular resistance that accompanies it—will be manifested under the fingers. The recoil, synchronized to this precise movement, will optimally resonate with all energetic rhythms of the organism, which will add extra value to our osteopathic normalization. It is an energetic phase that will act, in a controlled manner, softly and deeply on the tissular biorhythms of the bodily structure.

The Phase of Mentalization

Here the patient is asked to visualize the image of a personal problem that he or she wishes to treat (for example, the traumatic memory of the deaths of loved ones or of an accident, a repetitive nightmare, a stressful situation, etc.).

The protocol for this phase needs to be clearly explained to the subject because we need voluntary participation that is quite active. Once the phases of the recoil up to phase four have been set into motion, at the moment of apnea in inhalation or exhalation, the patient must visualize or mentally represent the problem to be dealt with. At this instant, the practitioner will feel a certain release of the lesion; then, after a few seconds, a new fascial barrier will form, as if the osteopathic lesion, because of the tension of the psychological stress, more strongly reappears. The adjustment will be done working at this maximum point of tissular resistance.

The Phase of Verbalization

This one follows the same principle as the previous one, except that instead of visualization the person will express his or her problem verbally.

Because it's impossible for someone to speak without breathing, we must start from phase two of the recoil and then we will let the patient verbalize his or her emotion. It is preferable to introduce the problem by a simple and open question, for instance, "How are you emotionally?" or "What do you think is the cause of your worries?" At this moment, if the osteopathic lesion is significant on the somatoemotional level, the action of putting the lesion under tension will provoke an interesting phenomenon. While the person is talking about a problem that touches him or her, the practitioner will notice very quickly that the speech and respiration will be modified, even to the point of a short apnea, while just at that instant the fascial barrier will clearly increase. At this precise instant, the patient's physical and psychological level are somehow connected, and the recoil will often be followed by a sigh, by tears, or by an autonomic system manifestation of emotional release.

Further Work on the Different Phases of the Recoil

These different experimental phases may be subject to further modification and improvement. With time and experience, practitioners can carry out their own research into integrating other parameters while working with fascial tension. Most important is not to lose sight of our goal: the maximum expression of the osteopathic lesion. With mastery of the principles and practice of the recoil, osteopaths have in their hands a very evolutionary technique for improving osteopathic adjustment.

The technical mechanics of the recoil that we have talked about, far from being different accessories, allow a real increase in the power of the corrective movement. In the same way that homeopathy has a progressive scale in the dilution of remedies, the different phases of the recoil offer the osteopath a possibility to modulate each treatment with precision. We can compare the different dilutions of the homeopathic remedies with the different phases of the recoil in the following way.

Phases one and two have a more physical action and cover a smaller territory. They are chosen for symptomatic targeting of a particular territory. Phases three and four cover a large number of biomechanical and metabolic factors of the total lesion and are longer lasting. Phase four is the one used most to adjust the primary and the dominant lesions. The experimental phases are used to orient the treatment towards a more subtle energetic or emotional release.

The different modalities of the recoil give more flexibility to the treatment, and they are not necessarily used in a linear step-by-step manner. For example, in certain cases we will first address the primary lesion with the phase four technique, and then work with the dominant lesion with a somatoemotional root using the experimental phases, then finish with symptomatic targeting work, using phase one or two techniques.

In general, the emotional phases of mentalisation or verbalization are not recommended for the first visit. It is preferable to come to know the patient better and first to rebalance the physical and energetic levels before we work on more subtle levels.

Sometimes it happens with phase four that work with a primary lesion doesn't result in much difference between inhalation and exhalation in amount of fascial resistance. It is then preferable to revert to phase two or to try the phase called tissular respiration, which integrates rhythms other than that of pulmonary respiration. This is because, since the principle of the recoil remains the same, it's possible to nuance each adjustment in order to adapt to all situations.

The Action Modes of the Recoil

The efficiency of the recoil is proven by the normalization of the mobility test and the clinical results that follow. The development of this technique has been based on practical work. But it is legitimate to try to rationally understand how physiologically a movement so simple and light can so easily release an osteopathic lesion. The scientific hypotheses that are most plausible relate to *neurological effects* and the *piezoelectric effect.*

Neurological Effects

Due to its high velocity and its very specific orientation, the impact of the recoil energetically stimulates the mechanoreceptors of Golgi, Ruffini, and Pacini, which are present in all fascial tissue. By means of an inhibitory reflex, the receptors of Golgi induce relaxation of the muscle that fixates the lesion. The receptors of Ruffini and Pacini will stimulate a reverse muscular contraction, which will release the tissular scarring that is at fault, and this will maintain the acquired correction. The recoil, by reprogramming the neurological aspect of the structure, will give it a more physiological position and function. This neurological effect is manifested the most where the mechanoreceptors are the most numerous, i.e. in the myofascial, articular, and visceral systems.

The Piezo Electrical Effect

The piezo electrical effect (from Greek *piezen:* "to press") is a physical phenomenon that, once we subject certain structures of a crystalline type to a specific pressure, will create at their surface an electrical polarization. The collagen fibers of the connective tissue, due to their semicrystalline nature, are biological material that is susceptible to this phenomenon. The pressure and the impulse of the recoil creates an electrical polarization that is susceptible to spreading on the surface and at a distance, and this would in part explain the neutralization of the secondary lesions that are often very far from the one that has been adjusted. It seems that the piezo electric effect is strongest in the bones, which would explain the incredible power of the recoil when it is applied with an intraosseous line of force.

Beyond the neurological and piezo electrical effects that we have talked about, other phenomena must also be taken into consideration. Quantum theory, the basis of modern physics, affirms that energy and matter have a similarly discontinuous structure. We can therefore predict that the impact of the recoil is enough to create corpuscular and undulatory modifications and waves in matter, a vibration effect that would also explain why after normalization we feel under our hands a much more fluid and light texture.

CHAPTER 7

The Spinal Unit

Global Examination

The spinal unit is the first functional unit we examine. For the sake of convenience, the patient is usually examined seated comfortably, leaving the spine in a position of articular neutrality. If circumstances require, the subject can be examined standing or lying prone.

By functional *spinal unit* we are referring to the occipito-vertebro-pelvic axis and the posterior thorax (costotransverse articulation). Even if the patient's primary lesion is located elsewhere in the body, we often have to treat a lesion of a vertebral segment as a dominant lesion or as part of symptomatic targeting work. We assume that readers are already familiar with the anatomy and biomechanics of the spine, and there is no need to review its importance in manual therapy. Thus, we will go on to describe how we test for lesions in this area.

The first thing we do is to test the mobility of each vertebral segment, one after the other, from the occiput to, and including, the coccyx. Global tests (described in Chapter 5) are carried out, with all concerned vertebral segments put under fascial and osteoarticular tension. We eliminate all active or passive mobilization of the vertebral spine so as not to modify or displace existing resistance. The other global tests follow each other very simply from the top to the bottom in the following order:

Figure 14
Spinal Unit A

Figure 15
Spinal Unit B

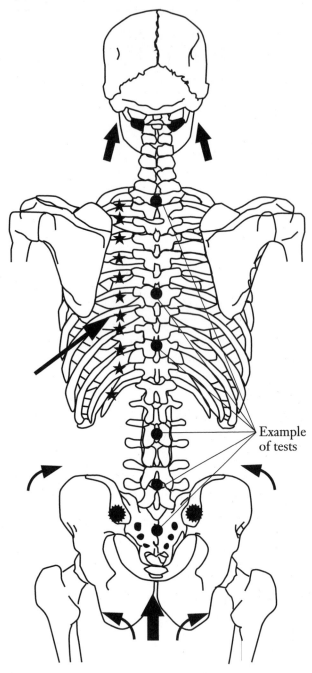

Example
of tests

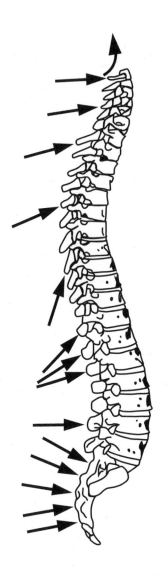

★ At the posterior rib angle
for the rib tests

● On the spinous process
for the vertebral tests

The Occipitoatlas Articulation

The occiput is tested by applying traction to the atlas (elevation upward), with both the practitioner's thumbs placed under the occiput squama. As with all symmetrical tests, we apply pressure and then accentuate right and left movements at the end points of the tension. If we feel blockage—a clear resistance under one of our thumbs—we will note the side of the fixation.

The Atlas Axis Articulation

The atlas is tested by combining posteroanterior pressure on the lateral mass and traction (elevation upward) to the axis. A tissular barrier that is manifested on the right or left indicates a fixation of the first cervical vertebra.

The Typical Vertebral Articulation

From C–2 down to and including L–5, we test the mobility of each vertebra by applying gentle pressure on the spinous process. This accurate global test will immediately indicate if there are segments in lesion, and each will be marked with a dermographic pen.

Both thumbs follow each other, alternately pressing, spinous process to spinous process, down the vertebral ladder. When the thumb that applies the pressure hits a barrier, we know there is a vertebral fixation; the normal state is when the spinous process gives no sensation of resistance. For the test to be accurate, it is important to respect the axis of the spinous process. Pressure must be applied with an orientation of posterior towards anterior but also with a slight oblique superior direction, depending on the vertebral level and the curve of the spine. All movements must be harmonious and ergonomic.

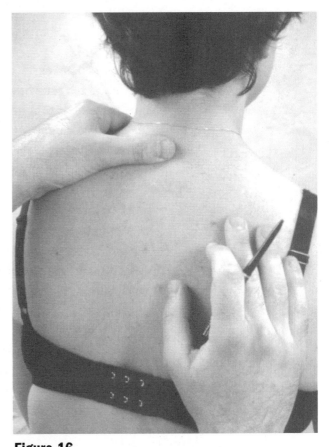

Figure 16

Global Test of C–7: The Left Hand Applies Posteroanterior Pressure on the Spinous Process of C–7

The Sacrum

As we have mentioned in our embryology review (Chapter 1), the sacrum must be considered as the fusion of five vertebrae. We therefore test the sacrum not globally but segmentally from S–1 to S–5, the same way we test the other vertebrae. It might be surprising that each sacral vertebra behaves on the functional level as a relatively independent biomechanical entity, but this is the way it works. Furthermore, a lesion of one sacral vertebra is a lot more significant than one of the whole sacrum.

We individually test each level of the sacrum by applying pressure on the tubercle, which corresponds to the median crest (fossil of the spinous process, S–1, S–2, S–3, S–4). At the level of S–5, the median crest has a bifurcation of spinous horns, which limits the sacral hiatus; the pressure test is applied directly on those two sacral horns. Just as when testing the other vertebrae, all fixations of an individual segment of the sacrum will be marked with a dermographic pen.

The Coccyx

This is a subcutaneous bone, easily accessible from the superior part of the gluteal fold. To test, with the right hand, palm facing up, we slightly lift the buttock of the patient (who remains sitting), so that the distal extremity of the third finger is in contact with the caudal extremity of the coccyx. From there, we apply light pressure upwards, to the axis of the coccyx, pressure to which we then add the components of side-bending right and left. We insist that the coccyx can be tested (and corrected) very easily externally, through the underwear, without need to touch the rectum. This allows us to approach the coccyx of all patients without exception, whatever their age, gender, or culture. As part of any general examination we must systematically test the coccyx. Lesions of these small bones are frequent and often have great consequences.

The Pelvis

The sacroiliac articulation is examined using two global tests. The first is applying posteroanterior pressure on the posterior superior iliac spine (PSIS). This test is symmetrical: done simultaneously on the right and left by applying a posteroanterior pressure with the thumbs on the ileum, in relation to the sacrum. Resistance indicates a posterior iliac lesion on the side that is blocked.

The second global test of sacroiliac articulation involves applying anteroposterior pressure on the anterior superior iliac spine (ASIS). This test is done symmetrically on the right and left, with the middle finger

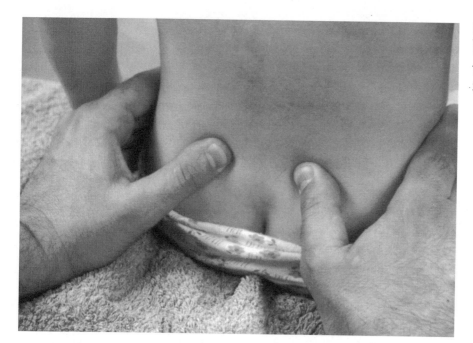

of each hand hooking at the ASIS and pushing the ileum in a posterior direction. Resistance indicates an anterior ileum lesion on the side of the restriction.

To these two global tests, we systematically add a test of the axis of the sacrum, a compression test of all three of its transverse axes. This can reveal any lesions due to diastasis of the iliosacral area, often associated with an intraosseous expansion lesion of the sacrum (discussed in greater detail later in the chapter). We test by applying convergent and symmetrical pressure with the two thumbs on either side of the PSIS, just behind the insertion of the gluteus medius. The pressure is applied at the level of S–1 for the superior transverse axis, at the level of S–2 for the middle transverse axis, and at the level of S–3 for the inferior transverse axis.

The Three Intraosseous Lines of Force of the Iliac Crest

Although they do not truly belong to the spinal unit, our examination of the osteoarticular part of the spine includes the following structures.

Using compression we test the external iliac line, the innominate line, and the iliac crest. The lesion along the intraosseous line of force of the ileum will often be pathogenic, with effects felt locally as well as at a distance. This type of lesion, classically ignored, is one of the most important discoveries that we have made in the last few years. (See Chapter 10.)

We also test the mobility of each rib, not by examining the major movement of inhalation and exhalation, but the minor movements at the costovertebral junction. A typical rib articulates in two distinct ways: its head with two successive vertebral bodies, and its tubercle with the corresponding transverse process. To test for lesions, we combine postero-anterior pressure at the costal angle (distraction of the costotransverse articulation) with lateral traction following the axis of the neck of the rib (distraction of the costovertebral articulation). We successively examine each pair of ribs from the 1st to the 12th, carefully respecting the angle of the rib. (The ribs become oriented more posterior and inferior as we move down the thoracic area.)

The particularity of the 1st, 11th, and 12th ribs, which each articulate only with one vertebra (instead of two), does not fundamentally change the test. All diagnosed restrictions at the level of the posterior thorax will be treated as seriously as those of the vertebrae and the pelvis, and will be marked on the patient with the dermographic pen.

Once the examination of the posterior aspects is finished, we start with the spine and use the balance test to compare all different vertebral fixations to find which are more severe (as described in Chapter 5). Although the balance test may be done in any order with the same results, we usually start by balancing the upper and the lower most lesions that have been found in the spine. We move away when one releases and stay in contact with the one that resists, continuing to balance that one with the next vertebral lesion. We proceed by successive elimination until we find the one dominant lesion of the spine.

We continue in the same manner to balance the fixations of the pelvis and those of the posterior thorax. We finish by balancing the dominant lesion of the spine against that of the pelvis and that of the ribs to identify the final dominant lesion of the occipito-vertebral-pelvic area.

Once the dominant lesion of the occipito-vertebro-pelvic and posterior thorax is found, the examination will continue, moving to other functional units (presented in the following chapters).

Treatment Protocol

Normally treatment is done with the patient in the same position as he or she was during the examination: sitting with his or her back to the practitioner. When we must act on a vertebral, pelvic, or costal lesion, whether as a primary, dominant, or symptomatic lesion, we proceed in the same manner: specific tests, adjustment (recoil), and verification.

Specific Tests

The specific tests of the articular segment to be treated allow us to identify the different degrees of restriction. For a typical vertebra, there are ten tests:

- flexion and extension;
- side-bending right and left;
- rotation right and left;
- lateral translation right and left;
- intervertebral decompression;
- line of force of the spinous process.

If many fixations exist, we will reduce the number to be addressed by using the balancing test, leaving only one parameter as the major one.

Adjustment

We will not review again the treatment by recoil that we have talked about in Chapter 6. But just as a reminder, the adjustment will be applied directly to the major tissular barrier that has been found in the specific test.

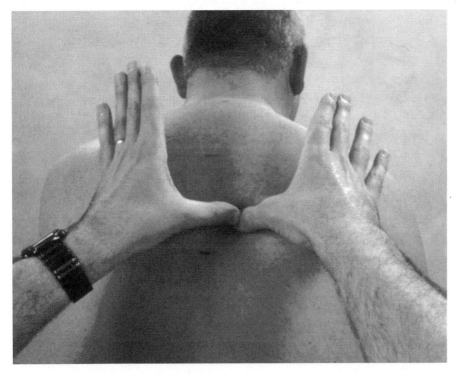

Figure 18.

Recoil Adjustment of a Right Posterior T–6

Verification

The immediate neutralization of a lesion is verified by repeating the global test: applying pressure on the spinous process. This test must come back normal. After we have liberated the dominant lesion of the spinal unit, we must then verify all vertebral, pelvic, and costal lesions that were marked with the dermographic pen. Note that normalization of a major restriction must totally or partially release all minor restrictions that are dependent on it.

If there are any lesions left, they will again be compared with each other by doing a balance test. The new dominant lesion that is found will be adjusted, or may be balanced against the dominant lesions of the other functional units.

Particular Situations in Treatment of the Spinal Unit

A corrective movement, just as the tests that preceded it, must remain totally pain free and without any real contraindication. This allows us to intervene even in critical cases of severe osteoporosis, of nonconsolidated fracture, of herniated disk, of postsurgery sequelae, with or without the presence of surgical material, of vertebral abnormalities, etc.

The treatment of the spine and the posterior thorax is always very short because the recoil technique takes only a few seconds. The efficiency of the recoil is immediate; the patient will generally feel better and results will last, if the total lesion has entirely been normalized.

The Coccyx

As we have said before, lesions here are frequent and their importance and seriousness should not be underestimated. If we have to normalize the coccyx, we ask the patient to lie on his or her side, with the lower extremities slightly bent. In this position, we will carry out the following specific tests, all externally, through the underwear:
- flexion and extension;
- side-bending right and left;
- rotation right and left;
- caudal traction (decompression of the sacrococcygeal articulation);
- cephalic pressure (intraosseous line of force).

Figure 19

Recoil Adjustment of a Left Lateral Flexion of the Coccyx (Side-Bending) with the Thumbs of the Right Hand

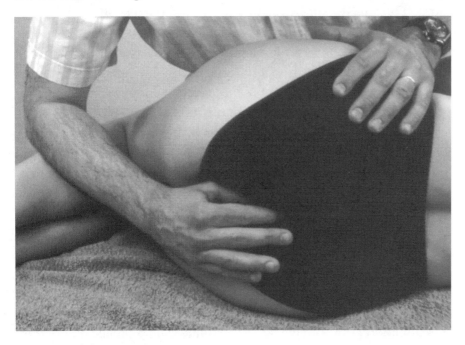

At times we must specially test one of the four or five coccygeal vertebrae, because intraosseous lesions are sometimes found in this area. We must remember that the coccygeal vertebrae only fuse together permanently after the fortieth year, and that the middle sacrococcygeal symphysis remains very mobile in pregnant women.

Once a maximal tension point of the coccyx is localized, we will apply the recoil in the usual manner: directly on it. The coccyx is an extremely sensitive territory, but the rapidity, the comfort, and the immediate efficiency of the recoil are very appreciated advantages of the technique.

Vertebral Abnormalities

Vertebral abnormalities can be located at any level, but statistically they are more common at the lumbosacral junction. The diagnostic is essentially carried out through radiology, but we don't buy in to the notion of "medical abnormality," meaning something untreatable.

Experience demonstrates that after osteopathic adjustment most vertebral abnormalities can be well tolerated. In all cases of spina bifida, asymmetry of the interspinous process articulation, lumbar fusion of S–1, or sacral fusion of L–5 (unilateral or bilateral, complete or incomplete), vertebral blockage acquired or congenital, spondylolisthesis, etc., we will use exactly the same test of tissular tension that we use on normal vertebra. The adjustment by recoil allows us to correct all articular and intraosseous lesions of any atypical spinal segment.

Spondylolisthesis, at the level of L–5, is caused by an anterior glide of the vertebral body in relation to the one below. The spondylolisthesis is generally due to the breakdown of the vertebral body and breaking apart of the superior articular process from the rest of the posterior arch, (or to the sliding of the posterior articular surfaces due to arthritis). The goal of an adjustment using the recoil technique on the spondylolisthesis is not reducing the displacement but neutralizing the anterior fixation that causes or maintains the positional imbalance. Osteopathic treatment will often improve the function of the segment in question.

In practice, we will approach the spondylolisthesis of L–5 through the abdomen, with the patient lying on his or her back, with the legs bent. Palpatory approach to this territory must be very cautious. Feeling the pulse of an artery under the fingers most likely indicates pressure on the bifurcation of the aorta located at the level of L–4. One most then move inferiorly to L–5. The recoil technique will be applied on the anterior surface of the vertebral body of L–5, which is more protruding in the case of spondylolisthesis.

The adjustment will be oriented in a posterior direction, towards the table and slightly superior, in the direction of the patient's head.

Herniated Disk

This well-known degenerative pathology of the intervertebral disk is mainly found at the level of the cervical and the lumbar spine. It usually causes neuralgia, due to the mass that pushes on the dura mater, or the root of the nerve. Not counting the important neurological conditions that necessitate surgical intervention, eighty percent of the neuralgia cases caused by discoradiculopathy respond quite well to osteopathic treatment. We do not recommend classical vertebral manipulation in the case of a herniated disk, but we do recommend the use of the recoil as a better way to act with efficiency and security on this type of lesion.

As is usual in the global process of Mechanical Link, we must first of all normalize the osteopathic lesions that are present in the subject. A herniated disk is only the presenting symptom, and we must examine the whole body to find the primary cause. Once we have generally rebalanced the body, it is then possible and advisable to symptomatically target the intervertebral joint that suffers. With a herniated disk, we often find a compression lesion of the vertebral tripod. We correct this lesion by means of a recoil treatment, with the goal of lifting the fixated vertebra away from the compressed disc. The specific adjustment usually brings rapid relief of sciatica, cruralgia, and other neuralgic pain that the patient suffers.

The Cervical Spine

Cervical lesions (except those at C–2 and C–7) are often an adaptation to a fixation elsewhere. It is therefore quite rare that we need to act at this level except for doing symptomatic target work. With the patient sitting down we can easily do all of our specific tests with one hand and use the other hand to stabilize the vertebrae below. The recoil technique is done in the same position, with one technical difference: after the adjustment, the second hand must immediately stabilize the cervical spine, in order to avoid the effect of whiplash.

Sacroiliac Diastasis

In spite of all the literature discussing the sacroiliac articulation, we think that the lesion known as *diastasis* has remained mostly ignored and mis-understood. Sacroiliac diastasis, in the osteopathic sense, is a very common situation: a functional lesion of the articular surface due to having received a traumatic or postural constraint of divergence. It's a mechanism similar to that of a sprain, where the articular surface has spread without a displacement of the bones. The sacroiliac then functions in articular misalignment, which, with time, will bring on articular instability in hypermobile subjects or an intraosseous expansion lesion of the sacrum in tight subjects.

The lesion of diastasis is generally increased by the classical type of articular manipulation that, in any case, the patient will say they don't hold. In fact, that type of manipulation usually serves to unblock the articular facets, as we can hear by the cracking that often follows this maneuver. And that's just what should *not* be done. This type of lesion must always be adjusted by means of compression in order to neutralize the peripheral tension that separates the articulation. To our knowledge the recoil is the only technique that can efficiently correct the lesion of diastasis. The recoil should be applied on the lateral side of the posterior superior iliac spine, in direction of the sacrum, and at the same level as the transverse axis implicated. The other hand will be placed on the opposite side as a counter support for the ilium.

Figure 20

Compression Test of the
Middle Transverse Axis
of the Sacrum (S–2)

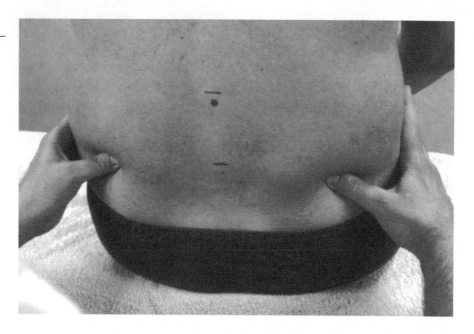

Here is a case study. Mr. A.M., thirty-five years old, was sent to us by his surgeon, who had operated on his herniated disk at the level of L–5-S–1. The patient complained of persistent lumbosacral pains on the right side, even following surgery (performed eight months earlier). He had received numerous manipulations and infiltrations but his pain was worsening. Upon postural examination, we noticed a protective position of the lumbar spine on the right side. The primary lesion turned out to be in the right knee, and the dominant lesion was a diastasis of the right sacroiliac on the middle transverse axis. After treatment the patient was seen one month later and found to have complete improvement and relief of the pain and total disappearance of the protective posture.

Atypical Lesions of the Iliac Bones

Since the iliac bones are part of the pelvis, it is easier to approach them when the patient is supine. For this reason, we include the atypical lesion test of the iliac bones in the protocol for examining the visceral pelvis.

The open iliac *(out-flare)* or closed iliac *(in-flare)* are articular lesions that often develop into osseous torsion of the iliac crest. The in-flare fixation is usually in relation to a visceral lesional chain, whereas the out-flare lesion relates to osteoarticular lesions of the lower extremities or of the spine. A well-done recoil usually releases the torsion of the ilium with ease and durability.

The superior ileum (up-slip) lesion is wrongly considered a traumatic lesion, when, most often, it is a postural lesion that starts out to have minimal effect but worsens rapidly. In fact, an ascending ileum, no matter what its initial cause, leads to a slightly shorter lower extremity. Since as bipeds we are programmed to lean on the shorter extremity, the ascension of the ileum will slowly but surely increase. The up-slip of the ileum is an *autoaggravating* lesion. The bone growth of a child with this excessive leaning will slow down (Delpech's Law). Therefore, the consequence of a superior ileum will be a false shorter leg (functional) evolving into a true shorter leg (anatomical) due to asymmetrical growth.

The up-slip ileum lesion is tested and corrected with the patient supine. By applying pressure on the iliac crest in the direction of the feet, we lower the ileum. The recoil adjustment of a superior ileum almost always allows us to lengthen the shorter leg by many millimeters. This rebalancing of the pelvis can be measured objectively by the difference between the tibial malleoli before and after the correction.

Summary—Working Principles

The spine, the pelvis, and the posterior thorax constitute a vast domain. Although we have touched upon only a few of the most important aspects, we have laid out a clear and coherent approach to this complex biomechanical unit. This approach is based upon several working principles:

- We must consider all existing articular and atypical intraosseous lesions.
- We must create a hierarchy of the different lesions that have been found during the examination and find the dominant one.
- We must compare the dominant lesion of the vertebral functional unit to the dominant lesions of the other functional units (osseous head, viscera, extremities, etc.).
- We must know how to efficiently, comfortably, and safely treat all vertebral, pelvic, and costal lesions that are primary or dominant.
- We must not intervene on a vertebral, pelvic, or costal lesion that is dependent on a primary lesion situated elsewhere. (Reasons for this are discussed later on.)

If we respect these general principles, treatment of the spinal unit will not give you any trouble. It will be efficient, quick, very precise and gentle on the patient.

CHAPTER 8

The Thoracic Unit

The Different Parts—Shell or Armor?

By *thoracic unit*, we are referring to the functional osteoarticular system of the thoracic cage. The name *thorax* comes from a Greek word meaning *shell*, and the thorax constitutes a protective wall for many vital organs such as the heart, the lungs, the liver, and the spleen. This capacity of protection depends on its solidity as well as its flexibility. However, since the anterior thorax is frequently exposed to physical trauma and greatly influenced by emotional stress, the natural flexibility of a living shell can be quickly replaced by the rigidity of a lifeless shell: our thorax becomes armor.

As we explained in the previous chapter, examination of the costovertebral articulation is more conveniently integrated with that of the spine. After work with the spinal unit, we move next to consider the anterior thorax. Since many fixations may exist here, it's not realistic or sufficient to do only a few global tests of the thorax. In the logic of Mechanical Link, we individually examine all structures susceptible to lesion, but treatment is not a daunting task. Using the balance test (see Chapter 5) we are able to find dominant lesion upon which the others depend, and address that.

In current practice, unless it's impossible, the patient will be examined supine with the practitioner standing on the right side of the patient.

Figure 21

Specific Test by Pressure
on the 2nd Sternebra

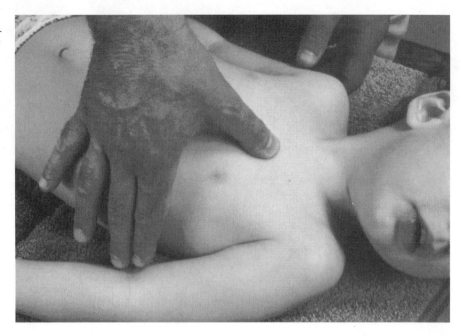

The Sternum

Just like the sacrum, the sternum is a bone made of different segments
that have been fused together. We individually test each sternebra as if
each were a separate biomechanical unit.

The tests are performed by directly applying pressure on each of
the seven sternebra, from the manubrium up to and including the xiphoid
process. Once we have completed these tests, we will have determined
each individual fixation participating in an intraosseous lesion of the
sternum.

The Sterno-Costo-Clavicular Joint

This is a very important joint: linking the scapular girdle to the sternum,
it has a function similar to that of the sacroiliac joint that links the pelvic
girdle to the sacrum. Although the sterno-costo-clavicular joint biomechanically belongs to the shoulder, it is functionally related to the thoracic unit and can be tested at this time. Due to its saddle-like articulation,
global tests must be done including two parameters, such as a posterior
pressure at the internal extremity of the clavicle, to which we add the
component of lateral traction.

The fixation of the sterno-costo-clavicular pivot is a common lesion.

Similar to torsion in the bones of the pelvis, we often find a clavicle in torsion with a paired fixation of both articulations, right and left. The balance test will allow us to determine which of the two sides is the dominant lesion. The diastasis lesion is also very common at this level

The Sternal-Costal Joint

The ribs, except for the last two floating ribs, are united to the sternum by the intermediary of the costal cartilage. Its flexibility allows for an increase of the thoracic diameter during inhalation Just as with any other connective tissue, if the costal cartilage becomes fixated, it is subject to formation of an osteopathic lesion in a process of symptoms we can recognize:

- inflammation—painful sensation of the cartilage under pressure;
- fibrosis—a noticeable loss of elasticity of the cartilage;
- sclerosis—visible calcification of the cartilage that can be seen on X-rays.

The more rigid the thoracic wall becomes, the more the pulmonary capacity will be decreased, and this has consequences:

- reduction of the gaseous exchange through the alveolo-capillary membrane;
- decrease of the level of oxygen in the blood;
- decrease of the alveolar macrophage activity and of the vibration of the hair of the pulmonary epithelium;
- increase in work of the cardiac pump.

Because structure governs function, the intervention of an osteopath to restore thoracic function—in which the costal cartilage plays a key part—is the determinant factor in preventing and healing respiratory or cardiovascular functional problems.

We individually test each section of costal cartilage using anterior posterior pressure. It is very important to properly access the first costal cartilage, which is very short and hidden under the clavicle, as well as costal cartilages 8, 9, and 10, which are a continuation of the 7th costal cartilage. (The 8th costal cartilage is an interesting anatomical landmark that is used to locate abdominal organs during the visceral examination.)

We complete the examination of the anterior thorax by specifically testing the costalchondral joint by applying anterior posterior pressure on the anterior extremity of the corresponding rib.

Diagnosis and Treatment

The series of pressure tests allows us to very rapidly identify all the elements of the thoracic cage that are restricted in mobility. For convenience, we mark all the lesions found with a demographic pen. If we find many lesions, which is very often the case, we must then follow global tests with balance tests that allow us to pinpoint the fixation that has the greatest tissular resistance: the dominant lesion of the anterior thorax.

We usually wait to begin treatment of any functional unit until all others are examined and their dominant lesions are found. Those are balanced against each other to find the primary lesion of the body. If the thoracic lesion ends up being primary, or one of the dominant ones to be treated, adjustment will be done directly on that structure. By applying the recoil following the principles given in Chapter 6, we can immediately liberate any thoracic blockage. This normalization can be verified: pressure tests will show a return to normal and a significant increase in the costal amplitude.

As with the spinal unit, the proper functioning of the thoracic unit impacts upon numerous organic and psychological functions, as shown in Figure 22.

Figure 22

The Impact of the Ribs on Organs and Psychological Functions

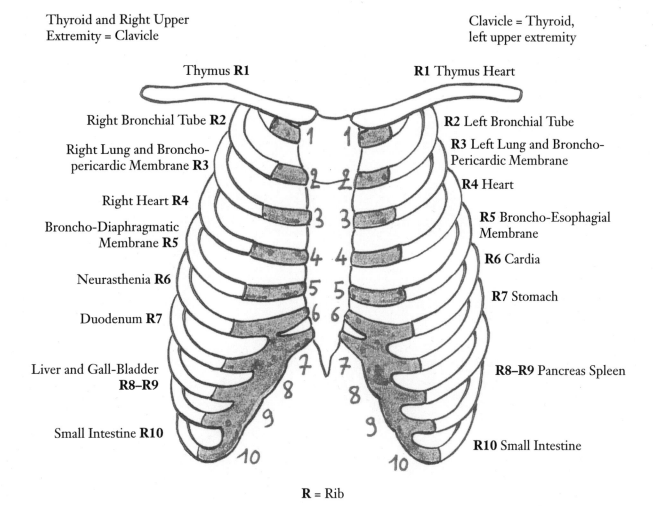

Thyroid and Right Upper Extremity = Clavicle

Clavicle = Thyroid, left upper extremity

Thymus **R1**

R1 Thymus Heart

Right Bronchial Tube **R2**

R2 Left Bronchial Tube

Right Lung and Broncho-pericardic Membrane **R3**

R3 Left Lung and Broncho-Pericardic Membrane

Right Heart **R4**

R4 Heart

Broncho-Diaphragmatic Membrane **R5**

R5 Broncho-Esophagial Membrane

Neurasthenia **R6**

R6 Cardia

Duodenum **R7**

R7 Stomach

Liver and Gall-Bladder **R8–R9**

R8–R9 Pancreas Spleen

Small Intestine **R10**

R10 Small Intestine

R = Rib

CHAPTER 9

The Extremities as a Functional Unit

Let's not amputate osteopathy by cutting off the possibility of fruitful work at the level of the extremities. In manual therapy, the osteoarticular system of the extremities is generally neglected, perhaps because it is considered the least noble functional unit, less essential than the spine, the cranium, or the viscera. However, if we underestimate the osteopathic importance of the extremities, we will only treat the articulation of an extremity for relief of symptoms, overlooking them as the possible site of most effective treatment for the whole organism.

Let us repeat with insistence, that the primary lesion—the one with the highest degree of tissular resistance, and the one that partly or totally inhibits a subject's functioning—is most often hidden. Therefore, it is not symptoms that must orient our osteopathic diagnosis but the complete and objective examination of all structures of the organism, including the upper and lower extremities, in search of the primary lesion.

Not all functional units of the body have the same biomechanical importance; however, we estimate that twenty to thirty percent of all primary lesions are located in the extremities. And if we add to this those related to the intraosseous lines of force and the arteries of the upper and lower extremities, we find the primary lesion in the geographical territory of the extremities in more than forty percent of all cases. This is a considerable number! So, let's not relegate working with the extremities to the fringes of osteopathy.

General Examination of the Extremities

As we have said many times, no matter why a subject consults us, a systematic and methodical general examination must be done. Since it would take far too long to examine the hundreds of possible lesions in the osteoarticular system of the extremities, we carry out a preliminary series of segmental global tests on both sides of the body. For the upper extremities, we test the hands and wrists; the forearms; the elbows; the arms; and the shoulders. For the lower extremities, we test the hips; the thighs; the knees; the lower legs; and the ankles and feet.

These global tests can be done equally well as pressure or traction tests. For convenience we prefer, if possible, to examine subjects lying in a supine position, with the upper extremities tested using traction and the lower extremities with the legs extended for traction tests or with legs flexed ninety degrees for pressure tests. Once completed, these global tests, requiring only twenty to thirty seconds in total, will have allowed us to identify all articular and osseous lesions of the extremities.

The general examination of the lower and upper extremities allows us a clear overview of the osteopathic organization of the patient at this level. It gives us the number and exact location of all individual lesions in the functional unit, and we simply need to balance them against one another to determine the one with the most tissular resistance: the dominant lesion of the extremities. After finishing the complete examination of the patient, this dominant lesion of the extremities will be balanced against the dominant lesions of the seven other functional units of the organism in order to find the primary lesion of the whole being.

If the primary lesion is found in the extremities, we must examine it in detail following the particular protocol for that articular or osseous unit. As we have already shown, the normalization of this primary lesion will lead to the liberation of all dependent secondary lesions in the lesional chain, whether these lesions are located in the functional extremities unit or elsewhere.

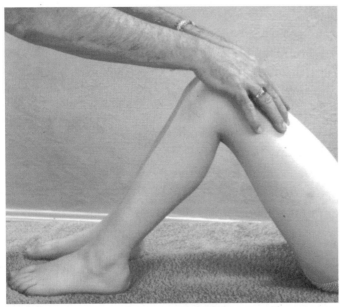

Figure 23

Global Test by Pressure on the Knees

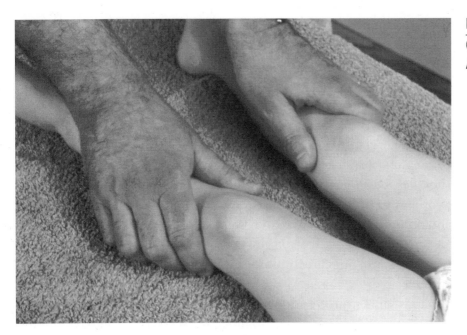

Figure 24

Global Test by Traction
Applied to the Knees

The Individual Articular Lesion

Before treating an individual articular lesion, we must analyze all its parameters of restrictive mobility, the sum of which creates sufficient fascial tension to fixate the articulation.

Each individual articular module is a complex entity consisting of many points of sub-unit articulation, with the exception of the hip, which has one coxofemoral articulation. To find the maximal fixation point of a lesion, we will proceed the way we'd use the zoom lens of a camera, and carry out specific tests of all parameters of the module in question.

For example, with a right shoulder individual lesion as primary or dominant, we would have four articular sub-units and two long bones to analyze:

- the sterno-costo-clavicular joint (six tests, as discussed in Chapter 8);
- the osseous segment of the clavicle (seven tests, as discussed in Chapter 9);
- the acromioclavicular articulation (nine tests, as discussed in Chapter 8);
- the osseous segment of the scapular spine (five tests, as discussed in Chapter 9 in the section on lesions of the long bones);

- the scapular thoracic articulation (five tests, as discussed in Chapter 9);
- the scapular humeral articulation (six tests, as discussed in Chapter 9).

Of these thirty-eight specific tests, (which would take too long to describe here) many will be positive. Many will correspond to one of the parameters of restriction that together add up to a global fixation of the shoulder. Balancing the different blockage points against one another allows us to find the most important one; for example, a lesion of the anterior humeral head. Once the osteopathic diagnosis is correctly established, the treatment is very simple: specific adjustment using the recoil technique, bringing directly posterior the humeral head, which is fixated anterior, in order to release the global shoulder.

This same protocol of specific test and normalization of the global lesion using the recoil will be applied, if necessary, on each of the following articular modules.

The Hand / Wrist

Made up of twenty-nine osseous pieces linked in a polyarticular chain, this module presents numerous lesional possibilities. In addition to the classical tests of minor movements of each element, analysis of this complex articulation must include the intraosseous test of the metacarpal and the specific tests concerned with opening and closing the wrist. This latter lesion that we frequently find in rheumatoid polyarthritis or in carpal tunnel syndrome is to be found there.

The Elbow

This is a largely underestimated articulation in manual therapy, most likely because a dominant lesion at this level tends to be locally asymptomatic, and so practitioners may not focus their attention on the area. However, it is a very important articulation that we systematically integrate into our protocol of examination, giving it the same attention as we do all the others so that we can make an accurate diagnosis.

This complex articulation has one synovial cavity, three distinct joints (humeroulnar articulation, radiohumeral, and proximal radioulnar articulation), and therefore, many specific tests must be carried out in order to examine it thoroughly.

The Shoulder

The shoulder is often the site of multiple traumatic and degenerative conditions for which an osteopath's intervention seems necessary, even essential. In functional anatomy, this module includes the sternoclavicular articulation, the acromion clavicular, scapular thoracic of the shoulder girdle, and the scapulohumeral articulation. A few points must be noted:

- The sterno-costo-clavicular articulation, a key articulation etymologically and in osteopathy, is tested individually in the examination of the anterior thorax (Chapter 8).
- The acromioclavicular articulation remains very important to analyze because numerous minor movements take place here, and it plays an important role in the function of the shoulder girdle.
- The coracoid process, with its numerous ligament and muscle attachments, is a crucial focus for many fixations of the scapula. It's the osseous landmark where most of the tests of the scapulothoracic articulation will be done.
- The scapulohumeral articulation is often the location of fixations, such as anteriority, superiority, or internal rotation of the humeral head. We also find impaction lesions following a fall in which someone bumps the shoulder, or retractile capsulitis and diastasis lesions in certain types of shoulder instability.

The Hip

Although it is a simple articulation (spherical type), the hip is very often not well understood; however, the frequency of progressive hip arthritis should be enough to push us to give it more attention. The restriction of mobility in internal or external rotation (myotension origin) is generally an adaptation and so there's little need to correct it. The principal fixations of the femoral head are mostly in expulsion, protrusion, and anteriority, and these are particular lesions that we should know how to test for and to adjust with good results. Finally, the obturator membrane (external sheath), in the context of the coxofemoral articulation, requires a specific examination.

The Knee

Because we use it so often in daily life, the knee articulation most often turns out to be the site of the primary lesion, and this is true no matter why our patients consult us. Thus, we use twenty-five specific tests to analyze in detail all three articulations: the femorotibial, the femoropatellar, and the tibiofibular. (Discussion of the possible intraosseous lesions at this level will be covered in Chapter 10).

We insist that the health problems of thousands of patients have been resolved after the knee has been treated. Most often, the lesion of the knee was primary but had no clinical symptoms.

The Foot/Ankle

In the architecture of an erect human body, the foot is the base of our static structure when we are standing, and the base of our dynamic structure when we are walking. Just as in a Roman church each stone is supportive, all osteopathic lesions of one element will be felt in the whole body.

Just like the spine, the foot provides a tripod support and is fundamentally essential for our posture. Just like the cranium, the foot consists of an internal, external, and transverse vault system, of which the muscles and the plantar aponeurosis represent the tie-rod.

The foot and ankle complex includes the talocrural articulation (ex tibiotarsal), the tarsal bone articulation, and the articulations of the forefoot (twenty-three distinct articulations for twenty-six osseous pieces). Each time the foot is a problem, we must know how to specifically analyze all the different elements. Here again, the efficiency of the osteopathic treatment depends upon the precision of the diagnosis.

Lesions of the Long Bones

Just by chance one day we noticed that the right and the left tibia of a person had different degrees of fascial tension; the pressure test done directly on the middle part of the bone gave us a soft and elastic tibia on one side of the body, while on the other it was rigid and hard. We were in the presence of another kind of osteopathic lesion, one not involving the restriction of mobility in an articular unit. Little suspecting just how far this discovery would take us, we adjusted the tibia by applying the recoil directly against the osseous resistance, and this had an immediate and surprising effect on the dynamics of the leg, giving it the same flexibility as on the normal side.

The tibia is the bone in the human body that receives the most shock over a lifetime (even if a person is not a soccer player!). However, the

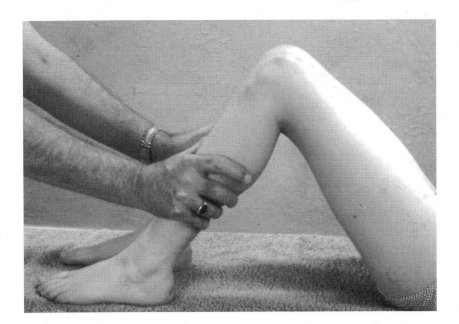

Figure 25

Global Test by Pressure
on the Tibia

frequency of intraosseous fixations of the tibia in the newborn surprised us. Most likely these are due to postural limitations related to the fetal position, imposing on this bone a certain curvature characteristic of a bowing lesion.

Excited by these findings, we decided to systematically test all our patients' long bones, which, just like the tibia, may be prone to this type of intraosseous fixation. We have found this type of lesion to be quite common, and it may be of traumatic or postural origin. In all cases, the rigidity of a long bone will have serious consequences for the mechanical behavior of the articulation above and below the segment.

If an intraosseous fixation is a factor in the lesional schematic, problems of extremities will not be resolved only by an articular approach. The biomechanics of the articular system depend upon the state of the skeleton, which is an expression of the fundamental principle of traditional osteopathy: *structure governs function.*

Once we have done the balance tests and determined that a long bone is the site of the dominant or primary lesion, we now have to determine precisely which of the parameters organizes this fixation. To analyze a long bone, we must do seven specific tests:

- internal and external bowing;
- anterior and posterior bowing;
- internal and external torsion;
- decompression (traction in the longitudinal axis).

Figure 26

Specific Test by Anterior
Bowing of the Right Tibia

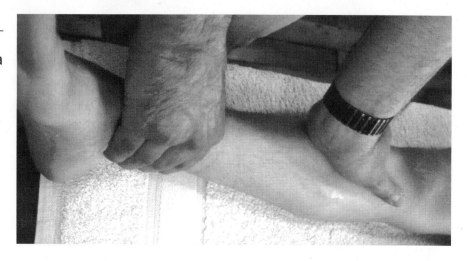

Once again, if we are in presence of multiple restrictions, we must balance them—in this case by stacking them—to find out which is the most important parameter of fixation: the one upon which we will have to act to regain the natural flexibility of this osseous segment.

The treatment is done by recoil, applying the adjustment directly against the tissular resistance of the bone. The normalization is immediately verified by global tests, which now should be negative and identical to results of tests of the healthy side.

All long bones of the extremities that have a fixation must be analyzed with the same protocol. This includes the clavicles, the humerus, the radius and the ulnar, the metacarpal bones, the femur, the tibia (and accessorily the fibula), and the metatarsal bones, as well as other bones or osseous segments that may be similar to a long bone, such as the spine of the scapula or the calcaneum.

The Articular Diastasis Lesion

This is a very particular type of osteopathic lesion that we have discovered and integrated into the protocol of Mechanical Link many years ago. It differs from orthopedic diastasis, where there is articular separation with rupture of the ligament. Here we're talking about the functional stages of a lesion where the articulation is blocked in a diverging position while preserving its anatomic integrity. Fascial tension maintains spread of the articular surface apart, and this, in time, leads to a reorganization of the bones themselves (shifting to accommodate the spreading of the tibia and of the fibula). That articular expansion leads to an intraosseous expansion that is the reason for chronic ankle sprains that never fully heal. The problem of articular expansion then becomes a problem of intraosseous expansion, as in the tissues of an old sprain that have never fully regained normal function.

Just as in articular diastasis, this intraosseous expansion corresponds to a transverse intraosseous line of force lesion: it is a failure of the osseous pieces to compress against one another.

A positive pressure test is the sign of a diastasis lesion (and of an intraosseous expansion lesion that will follow it over time). The tension test for the articular diastasis is to compress the osseous pieces against one another. A positive test, i.e. the rigidity of the articulation transversely, reveals a failure of articular convergence (diastasis lesion) with or without intraosseous expansion associated with it.

A functional diastasis lesion often leads to hypermobility of the articulation. The global test of the functional unit may be negative, so the diagnosis of diastasis is difficult during the general evaluation of the extremities. Therefore, testing for articular diastasis and of its slow evolution into an intraosseous lesion is not included in the general evaluation of the articulation of the extremities. Instead we look for this during testing of a different functional unit: that of the intraosseous line of force (Chapter 10).

The articular diastasis and the intraosseous expansion lesion are difficult to correct with classical techniques. The worst choice would be a thrust type of manipulation, which, contrary to its intention, often increases the instability of the diastasis. The aim is to bring the articular surfaces closer. Fortunately, applying the recoil directly against the tissular resistance allows us to very easily reduce this lesion of diastasis as well as the intraosseous expansion lesion.

In the upper and lower extremities we find diastasis lesions of the articulation such as the following:
- distal radioulnar articulation;
- proximal radioulnar articulation;
- sterno-costo-clavicular articulation;
- acromioclavicular articulation;
- distal tibiofibular articulation (most often following a lateral sprain of the ankle;
- proximal tibiofibular articulation.

At the level of the pelvis, we also find the diastasis lesion of the sacroiliac articulation, and diastasis of the symphysis pubis, often seen on women who have had children.

The lesion of diastasis is certainly one of the most pernicious lesions because it is little known, poorly understood, and difficult to approach with the usual techniques of manual therapy. With Mechanical Link, we are not only able to make a strong case for the reality of this type of osteopathic lesion, but we also give the practitioner techniques to easily diagnose (pressure test) and correct (recoil) it.

Symptomatic Lesions "Not to Treat"

Certain individual articular units may show one or more clinical symptoms (pain and functional difficulty, etc.) even though the global tension tests are negative. This situation is not so puzzling as it might seem, because it simply corresponds to a hypermobility of the segment in question. Whatever the cause, an excess of movement in an articular structure affects the articulation's mechanics just as much as a fixation of the same structure. So, obviously, all minor mobilization or strong manipulation of a hypermobile segment would just aggravate the problem. In osteopathy, we should never treat a structure that is not fixated, even if that's the reason the patient came for treatment, and he or she insists. We must not be blinded by the symptom but look for the cause. Generally, a hypermobile segment is compensating for one or many restrictions situated elsewhere. By adjusting a primary or a dominant lesion where it is found, we will rapidly and efficiently relieve the hypermobility in the articular unit without having to work on it directly.

Symptomatic Lesions "To Treat"

In certain cases when its minor movements are analyzed, an osteoarticular unit with negative global test results may be found to have one or many parameters of restriction of mobility. This situation is noticeable in acute cases and in recent cases because the lesional schematic will not yet have had time to take place. For example, with a recent ankle or knee sprain, the global tests of the articulation are often negative. A sprain that is limited to the inflammatory stage will not create a sufficient fascial lesion to block the articular unit. However, even if they're not important enough to fixate the whole of the segment (and therefore participate in the total osteopathic lesion), these restrictions may have a sufficient painful effect to disturb the local biomechanics, and thus we should treat them.

The treatment of acute and recent lesions follows two different protocols: normalization of the dominant lesion of the extremities functional unit; and symptomatic adjustment of all minor lesions of the affected segment. So, for an acute right ankle sprain (for which the global test results are negative,) we start the treatment by neutralizing the one or many dominant lesions of the extremities, for example the left knee, then the right hip, so that the entire functional unit has been normalized. Once the global balancing is attained, we can focus our therapeutic action on the sprain by adjusting all minor restrictions of the foot and ankle area. (The protocol for this treatment is presented in Chapter 15, on particular therapeutic orientations).

This symptomatic intervention, although it stays localized to the individual unit concerned, will have a rapid effect that is particularly appreciated in certain circumstances. But, just as with cars emergency repairs never replace general maintenance and repair, the necessity to address symptoms directly at times should never cause us to lose sight of the global nature of the osteopathic treatment.

10

The Unit of the Intraosseous Line of Force

The Human Body—From Biomechanics to Tectonic Architecture

The osteopathic lesion may be defined as a restriction of mobility of a structure in the organism: restriction of mobility caused and maintained by an abnormal resistance of the connective tissue. The connective tissue is the only tissue of the human body that may scar (inflammation—fibrosis—sclerosis), and it is at this level—the level of the fascial barrier—that scars, lesions, and adhesions are found that may limit and restrain movement.

Embryology teaches us the central role of the connective tissue, which evolved from the mesoderm. This mesoderm—the intermediary and central tissue—unifies and links all the elements of the organism. It is the osteopathic mechanical link. Since they share a common embryological origin, the osseous system must be addressed in the same way as all other connective tissue in the body.

Classical osteopathy essentially focuses on the articular, in the sense that it is mainly interested in the mobility between two anatomical parts. Whether it is peripheral or vertebral skeletal articulation, a cranial suture or visceral gliding, this focus always involves the junction of two elements and not the tissular quality of the element in question. However, in the last few years of systematic research and work in Mechanical Link, testing fascial resistance zones using our tension tests has enabled us to discover fixations that have not been described up to now, notably those concerned with the transverse and longitudinal osseous system—*lines of force*.

Figure 27

Intraosseous Lines of Force: External, Intermediary, Internal

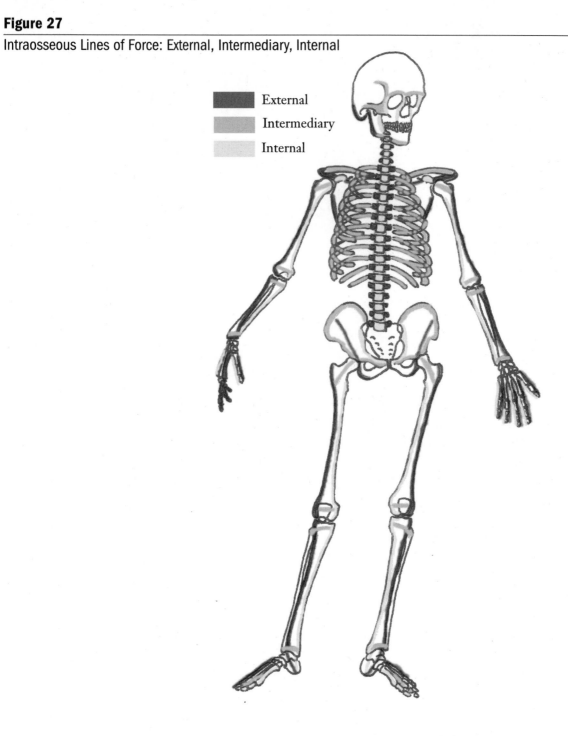

Once we had uncovered evidence for the intraosseous line of force—the real supporting beam of the skeleton—we were required to reconsider the way we look at this structure and to approach the architecture (organization, structure) of the body in a different, more complete, way. In fact, we had to go beyond the classical osteopathic mechanical model and to look at a tectonic architectural model.

In the biomechanical model, minor articular movements govern the major articular movements. (This is the difference and interest of osteopathy compared to physical therapy). However, Mechanical Link being based on the fundamental principle of A.T. Still's osteopathy, which states that structure governs function, we therefore propose this: that *the intraosseous lines of force govern minor movements* (and thus all major movement).

Let's use a simple example to explain. If the opening and closing of a door represents the major movement, the biomechanical model would consider that the minor articular movement of the hinges is responsible for this major movement. So if the door is stuck, the aim of the osteopath would be to restore normal articular play at the hinges in order to improve the door's opening and closing. However, in Mechanical Link we want to look more deeply. We might suspect that the vertical frame of the door is sagging or warped, which will also interfere with the movement of the door. To work only on the hinges will not solve the problem. We consider that this vertical structure constitutes the true axis of movement and represents the line of force upon which we must act to restore both the minor movement and the major movement of the system.

Anatomically, the lines of force are an objective reality: they act as reinforcement within the osseous structure where there are important constraints (stress). These intraosseous lines of force have nothing to do with the line of gravity of Little John. The intraosseous lines of force are mostly constituted of the cortical of the compact bones, and follow the trabeculae, where they spread out like a fan. The cortical of the bone has the function of *transmitting* stress, and the spongy bone has the function of *absorbing and spreading* stress.

In an architectural model of the osseous system, we can say that the skeleton consists of different structural components:

- The *pillars* are the supportive vertical structures such as the tibia, the femur, the spine, the ascending branch of the mandible, the mastoid, and so on.
- The *beams* are the supportive horizontal structures such as the calcaneum, the tibial plateau, the horizontal branch of the mandible, the petrous portion of the temporal bone, etc.
- The *flying buttresses are* external structures, such as the fibula, the clavicle, the scapular spine, and the zygomatic arch of the temporal bone, that provide equilibrium.
- The *arches* are semicircular structures such as the neck of the femur, the curved line of the ileum, the iliac crest, the ribs, the curved line of the temporal bone in the cranium.

- *Vaults* are structures such as the plantar vault, the parietal vault, the occipital vault, and the frontal vault.
- The *keystones* are structures such as the second cuneiform at the level of the foot, S–2 at the level of the sacrum, or the bregma (anterior fontanel) at the level of the cranium.

The different lines of force are linked to one another, either directly by an articulation (e.g. the scapular spine and the clavicles; the tibia and femur) or by the fascia or the muscle that extends from it (e.g. the iliopsoas, which links the internal line of force of the femur to the arch of the ilium).

At points along these intraosseous lines of force, it is not uncommon to find calcification that will reinforce the connective, ligamentous, or tendinous tissue if excessive stress is placed upon the area. Thus, for example, the calcification of the supraspinatus tendon prolongates the external line of force of the humerus; and the calcification of the transverse ligament of the scapula prolongates the line of force of the coracoid.

When an intraosseous line of force is fixated, the bone loses its capacity to diffuse or spread out the impact of stress. This type of blockage forces an articular system to act repetitively as a piston, and this in turn has a destructive effect that leads first to pain, and then to a more and more marked degeneration of the articular parts themselves. Such a blockage at an intraosseous line of force may mark beginning of a process leading to arthritis.

The Physiology of the Bones

Bone is a viable tissue that has many functions. Although it seems inert, actually, our skeleton is constantly active and has several important functions:

- Metabolic Function—Osseous tissue contains an immense reservoir of phosphorus, magnesium, sulfur, potassium, and especially calcium. These must be held in readiness for use to maintain constant blood level (homeostasis) and to supply other parts of the body with the minerals they need. The adipose cells in the yellow marrow of the bones are also a storage place for reserves of energy.
- Hematopoetic and Lymphatic Function—The red marrow, mostly located in the epiphysis, is the connective tissue that produces blood cells (red blood cells, white blood cells, and platelets).
- Mechanical Role—The osseous system supports and protects the soft

tissues, at the same time allowing movement. To do so, the bone must remain solid and support all kinds of stress (pressure, traction, torsion) without breaking. This remarkable resistance of our skeletons represents an ingenious compromise between rigidity and malleability; the bone must be well mineralized but should also be flexible and compressible.

Working with the Intraosseous Lines of Force

All intraosseous lines of force form a network that travels without interruption throughout the entire body and constitutes in itself a functional unit. The particular examination of these lines of force is always integrated into the general osteopathic examination that we practice. We directly test these lines of force by putting them under tension (compression) in the longitudinal axis. This pressure test must be done with counterforce at opposite ends of the bone. Resistance to this pressure, which will be felt under the finger as a blockage, indicates a lesion.

We systematically test the principal lines of force of the skeleton, for instance, the external and internal longitudinal line of force in the long bones; the transverse line of force in the epiphysis. We test for articular diastasis and its evolution into an expansion lesion of the intraosseous line of force. There are numerous possibilities for lesions in this functional unit of the intraosseous line of force.

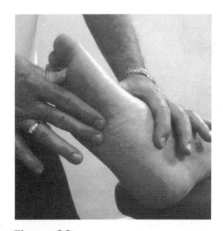

Figure 28

Intraosseous Compression Test of the 2nd Metatarsal of the Right Foot

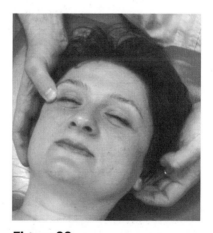

Figure 29

Intraosseous Compression Test of the Right Frontal to Left Temporal Beam

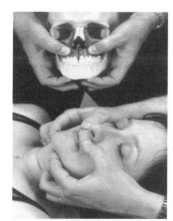

Figure 30

Intraosseous Compression Test of the Canines (Teeth 13–43 and 23–33)

The Lines of Force of the Extremities

These directly correspond with the acupuncture meridians, which is empirically confirmed by the work of E. Voll and by our clinical experience. For instance, Mr. S.N., thirty-seven years old, suffered from recent cephalagia, and came to see us. Examination revealed that the line of force of the fourth metatarsal of the left foot (gall bladder meridian) was a primary lesion, so we knew that adjustment at this line of force should release all other lesions. One hour after this treatment, Mr. S.N. felt great fatigue that forced him to lie down, and also nausea and nervousness. Two hours after these reactions, he felt just fine, and his headaches were gone and did not come back.

Figure 31

Lines of Force of the Legs/Feet
From R. Voll

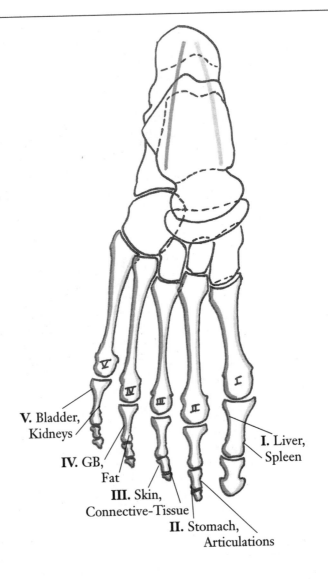

V. Bladder,
Kidneys

IV. GB,
Fat

III. Skin,
Connective-Tissue

II. Stomach,
Articulations

I. Liver,
Spleen

The Lines of Force of the Arms, Legs, and Shoulder Girdle

Mrs. C.B., seventy-two years old, consulted us for scapulohumeral degenerative arthritis, an extremely debilitating illness from which she had suffered for more than twenty years, in spite of medical and physical therapy treatments. In her X-rays we could see a thickening of the external cortical of the humerus, and during examination, we found that the external line of force of the humerus was very rigid. Our intervention was limited to a single adjustment of this lesion. To our great surprise, when Mrs. C.B. came for reevaluation a month later we could see a spectacular improvement in function: she was nearly free of pain and able to elevate her arms easily. Subsequent treatments continued to improve this result.

Figure 32

Lines of Force of the Arms/Hands

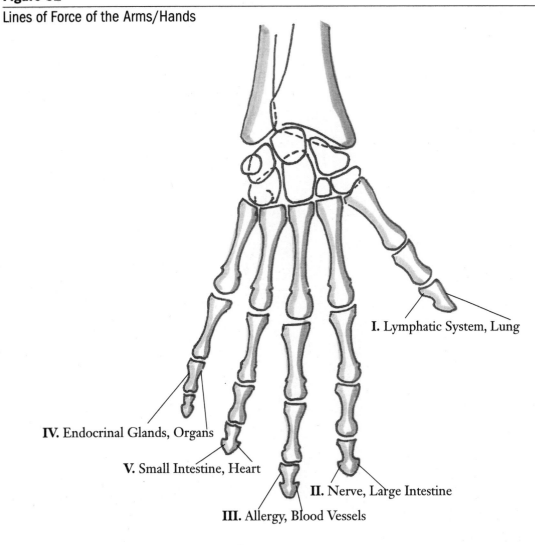

I. Lymphatic System, Lung

IV. Endocrinal Glands, Organs

V. Small Intestine, Heart

II. Nerve, Large Intestine

III. Allergy, Blood Vessels

The Lines of Force of the Osseous Head

These play a major role in many pathologies (fatigue, depression, vertigo, headaches, tinnitus, etc.). One very special case is the line of force of the teeth. Our work not only demonstrates that this particular lesion has a direct influence on occlusion, but it also has a reflexive action on the overall functioning of the organism, a correspondence also established by Voll. We are currently investigating, with promising results, the relationship between the dental lines of force and the visceral system.

Here is an interesting case that illustrates. Mrs. B.F. complained of numbness to both forearms and both hands, especially noticeable at night. The symptoms had appeared six months earlier, and greatly interfered with her sleeping. In the previous two years she had also suffered episodes of right dorsal pain. All medical examinations proved negative, with the exception of an ultrasound, which showed a slightly enlarged liver.

Osteopathic evaluation revealed a primary lesion in the dental line of force of the right superior canine (tooth 13), and Mrs. B.F. told us that

Figure 33

Architecture of the Osseous Head

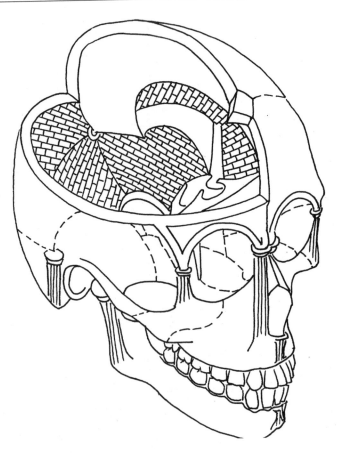

Figure 34

Lines of Force of the Osseous Head

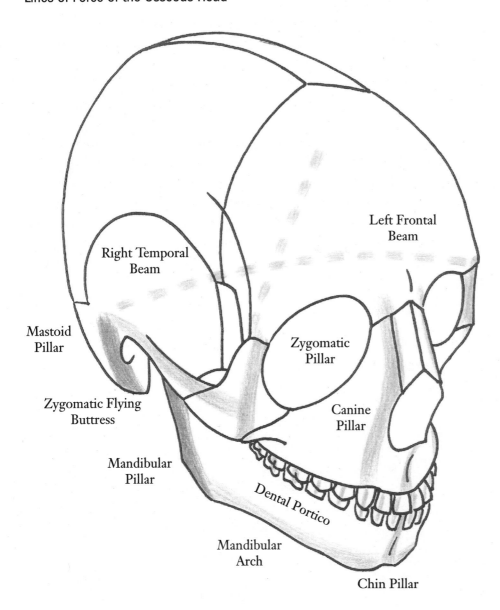

Left Frontal
Beam

Right Temporal
Beam

Mastoid
Pillar

Zygomatic
Pillar

Zygomatic Flying
Buttress

Canine
Pillar

Mandibular
Pillar

Dental Portico

Mandibular
Arch

Chin Pillar

she had needed dental work on that tooth about a month earlier. According to Voll, tooth 13 corresponds to the liver. Our osteopathic treatment first addressed this dental line of force, and second, T–2 (the second thoracic vertebra, which was fixated in right translation). A month later, Mrs. B.F. told us that all numbness had disappeared and the right dorsal pain was gone.

The Lines of Force of the Spine

The spine is a flexible stack of tripod-like segments. The architectural organization of the osseous trabeculation transmits and disperses the stress of the pressure on the anterior pillar (disk and vertebral body) and on the posterior pillars (the articular facets). This trabecular system extends to the spinous process. By testing the spinous process with pressure, we are able to determine the capacity of each vertebral segment to spread out the stress.

Some vertebral restrictions persist in spite of articular correction that was well done. These rebellious vertebral fixations often correspond to lesions of the intraosseous line of force, lesions that are easily released with a recoil adjustment to the axis of the spinous process. Normalization of this very frequent lesion of the spinal line of force allows the spine to regain better mechanical adaptation to the external load and body weight that it must bear and adjust to.

Figure 35

Intraosseous Lines of Force of the Pelvis

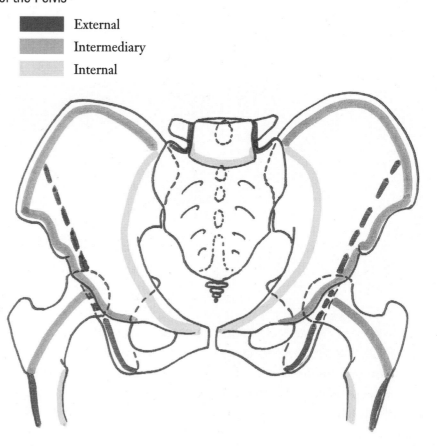

■ External
■ Intermediary
■ Internal

The line of force of the coccyx deserves particular attention. Support of posterior articulation is transmitted through the line of force of the pelvis, but this connection is indirect, transmitted by the intermediary of the sacroiliac joints. Only the line of force of the coccyx is directly connected to the vertebral axis. As long as blockage in the line of force of the coccyx is not treated, our vertebral treatment cannot be successful and complete.

Examination and Treatment Protocol

After all the fixations found on functional lines of force units have been tested for and found, these will then be balanced against one another to determine the dominant lesion. The dominant lesion of the intraosseous lines of force will be systematically integrated with the total lesion and then balanced against the other osteopathic fixations that were found. As we have said before, this procedure allows us to establish precisely which one is the primary lesion.

If the blockage in one of these lines of force ends up being primary or dominant, we will then liberate the intraosseous structure with our usual technique of recoil. Once the adjustment has been done, we will test to verify that the intraosseous line of force has reestablished its normal compressibility.

The normalization of an intraosseous line of force will have consequences at three levels:

- **Local**—For example, normalization of the movement of the knee and the hip by an adjustment of the external line of force of the femur.
- **Distant**—Adjustment will immediately liberate all secondary lesions that depend on it, no matter where they are found.
- **Deep and General**—Adjustment will mobilize the energy that was blocked.

The energetic impact of these lines of force is often remarkable, and sometimes surprising. It's not forbidden to think—even if we need to prove this objectively—that by addressing them we can have a significant impact on the most important functions of the bones: the metabolism of calcium and hematopoesis.

A Particular Case—Blockage
of a Cranial Ossification Center

Blockage in the cranial ossification center seems to be a special and interesting case concerning the lines of force. Detailed examination of the cranium allows us to discover resistance in the frontal, parietal, and occipital ossification centers. These represent the ossification centers of the cranial vault, which have a membranous origin. Blockage of a cranial ossification center is manifested by a significant rigidity during the pressure test.

A primary or dominant fixation of a cranial ossification center seems to correspond to a psychological disturbance. The frontal ossification center relates to mental fixation—fixed ideas that are never changed or resolved, decisions that are not made, constant preoccupation. The parietal line of force relates to emotional disturbance—moodiness, behavioral troubles of a child, irritability, or cyclothymic sadness. The occipital ossification center relates to instinctual behaviors. The ossification center on the left side corresponds to a more recent problem, most often related to an event, generally consciously known by the patient, whereas on the right side the concern is a deeper problem and unconscious.

An adjustment by recoil of a predetermined fixation at the level of the cranial ossification centers instantaneously normalizes the blockage at that point and liberates the imprinted stress at that level. This makes it possible for the patient to establish better physical and psychological equilibrium. Our action on the somatoemotional level may be reinforced by using the experimental phases of the recoil (mentalisation or verbalization of the problem, described in Chapter 6).

In all cases, osteopathic treatment must refer to and be supported by knowledge of the osseous structure, even when it is addressing the more subtle levels. In order to treat more than just the structure we must look inside rather than outside of the structure.

"Arthropath" or Osteopath?

The discovery of the intraosseous lines of force and their strong impact within the total lesion represents a giant step forward for osteopathy. By taking into account this type of lesion, practitioners may resolve many pathologies through manual therapy. Integrating the intraosseous lines of force into the work allows it to surpass the limits of the articular and really penetrate into the world of osteopathy. Without any doubt there is much more to be discovered: as A.T. Still said, "the study of a bone in its totality would require an eternity."

11

The Visceral Unit

A Return to the Basics

T he osteopathy that came to us via England was essentially an articular approach to the spine, and during our training we did not real-
ize how much emphasis, A.T. Still, the founder of our art, had put on the
visceral system. Through reading Still and his direct disciples, such as
E.W. Goetz, we learned that many techniques involving manipulation of
the organs (liver, stomach, intestines, ovaries) were routinely practiced by
the first American osteopaths. However, in France, we had to wait for the
work of J.P. Barral to bring the viscera back to their rightful place as part
of the total lesion, so dear to us.

In Mechanical Link, we consider the visceral unit to be just as important as all other functional units of the organism. Since it behaves biomechanically very similarly to the units in the osteoarticular system that
we are already familiar with, the visceral unit reacts very well to the techniques of Mechanical Link.

Examination Protocol

Most components of the visceral system are of mesodermic origin, including the different fascial envelopes of the organs, the ligamentous system
which supports them, the serous, muscular, and mucus tunica of the
viscera, as well as some organs, such as the heart, the spleen, and the kidneys, which have all the same osteopathic characteristics as other con-

nective tissue. Because the pathological process that leads to their scarring is identical, an osteopathic lesion, whether of one of the body's hard elements, such as the bone, or of a soft element, such as the viscera, will be translated into tissular resistance that we will feel during our tension tests.

We examine the visceral unit with the patient supine, arms alongside the body with the legs straight; and preferably, the practitioner stands on the right side of the table, even if left-handed. We carry out the test by using our hands to apply a combination of pressure and traction on the fascia of the viscera.

The tests proceed like this. First, by applying soft and progressive pressure on the topographic zone of the viscera to be tested, we create global tension on the whole tissular environment. Second, by applying traction from a mobile point in relation to a fixed point we focus this tension of the fascial structure on a very precise element of the viscera in question. A practitioner needs thorough knowledge of the anatomy of the organs to be tested and a lot of practice to be able to execute these tests with the required precision and subtlety.

We approach the visceral unit starting with the superficial (the empty viscera) and proceeding to the deep (the full organs). We examine them one after the other: working with the fascial structure of the digestive tract, the pelvis, the urogenital organs, the pancreas, the spleen, the liver, and then the respiratory and cardiac system. An experienced practitioner can carry out the tests quickly and smoothly, which allows for a detailed examination of the entire visceral unit—including diagnosis of the dominant lesion—in four or five minutes. The number of tests need not be daunting!

The Viscerocutaneous Depressions

Experience and a good knowledge of anatomy enable recognition of the palpatory landmarks of the different organs. To facilitate this search we have established a technique that uses the superficial cutaneous depressions, which allows us to palpate most corresponding visceral structures with precision.

The visceral mass is neither homogenous nor uniform; the contours of the superficial fasciae are closely related to those of the deep fasciae. We can therefore locate an organ by its parietal topography. By letting the hand glide very superficially, following certain anatomic landmarks, with a certain orientation, we will find the underlying organ and its form and

Figure 36

Main Abdominal Cutaneous Dip (Depression)

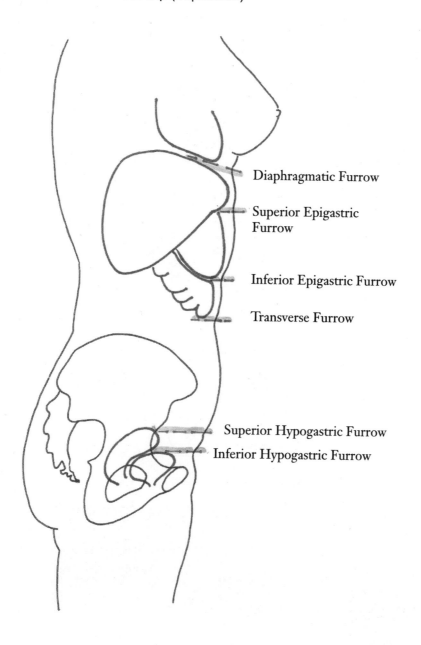

Diaphragmatic Furrow

Superior Epigastric Furrow

Inferior Epigastric Furrow

Transverse Furrow

Superior Hypogastric Furrow

Inferior Hypogastric Furrow

position. Not only are we able to delimitate the location of the visceral structure following its superficial tissular contours, but we use these viscerocutaneous depressions as direct access to the organs to be tested.

As we teach it, this superficial palpation of the cutaneous contours can be used on other anatomic structures of the human body.

Figure 37

Main Abdominal Cutaneous Dip (Depression) Front View

1. Diaphragmatic Furrow
2. Superior Epigastric Furrow
3. Mesenteric Furrow
4. Inferior Epigastric Furrow
5. Transverse Furrow
6. Ceacel Furrow
7. Sigmoid Furrow
8. Superior Hypogastric Furrow
9. Inferior Hypogastric Furrow
10. Iliac Furrow
11. Trochanter Furrow
12. Renal Furrow

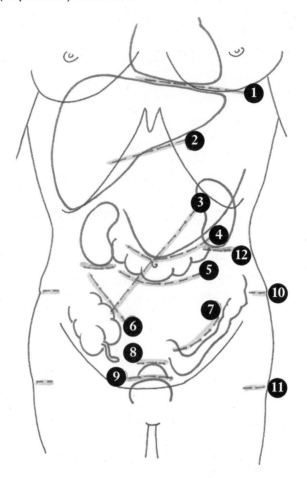

Figure 38

Locating the Inferior Border of the Transverse Colon

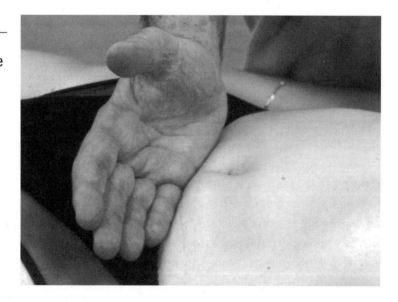

The Digestive Tract

We work with the digestive tract from the mouth to the rectum.

The Buccal Floor

The buccal floor is a true diaphragm, consisting of the extrinsic muscles of the tongue and the fasciae that line it, and continuing in the neck, with the subhyoid muscles and the superficial cervical aponeurosis. We test the buccal floor by applying pressure cephalically, towards the root of the tongue.

The Pharynx

This structure is the juncture of the digestive tract and the airways; it is used for swallowing, but also participates in the processes of breathing and speaking. We essentially test its accessible area, which is the oropharynx, by tractioning caudally.

The Cervical Esophagus

Located behind the trachea, anterior to the spine, we have access to the esophagus at the anterolateral portion of the neck, making sure to push slightly lateral in order not to compress the carotid artery or the jugular vein. The test is mostly done using longitudinal traction.

The left side of the cervical esophagus is more often in lesion than the right side, probably because of tension from the stomach on that side.

The Thoracic Esophagus

Located in the posterior mediastinum, the thoracic esophagus is between the heart and the thoracic spine, impossible to access directly. To test we apply traction between the two extremities of that portion of the esophagus.

This is a common lesion in the newborn, and it is a factor in the regurgitation often present in the first few months of life.

The Abdominal Esophagus

This short end portion of the esophagus deserves special attention. We access it by going down deeply at the 7th costal cartilage on the left, and test it by applying pressure-traction with both thumbs. A spasm of the abdominal esophagus is often related to the first stage of upper stomach suffering.

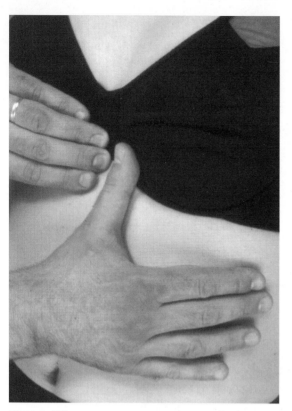

Figure 39

Test of the Cardia

The Cardia

We test this juncture of the esophagus and stomach, working through the thoracic cage, and pushing lateral the fundus of the stomach. This test allows us to evaluate the closing of the gastro-esophageal valve against the lesser curvature of the stomach.

A fixation at this level is the second stage of pathomechanical conflict in this territory, and the patient often complaints of acid reflux.

The Fundus

We test the superior part of the stomach by applying traction caudally.

A thoracic fixation of the stomach corresponds to the third stage in the lesion of the cardio-esophago-fundus junction. The patient may suffer from pyrosis, thoracic compression with apnea, cardiac palpitations, or repeated coughing. It is often the location of the hiatal hernia, a pathology we can often treat with good results.

The Body of the Stomach

The form, situation, and dimension of people's stomachs greatly vary, but we must first of all topographically locate this organ on the patient. To properly examine the stomach we must do few specific tests:

- three tests of the attachments (ligaments);
- three tests of mobility;
- three tests of the structure of the stomach.

A fixation of the phrenicogastric ligament, a restriction of the pendular mobility of the stomach, or a spasm of the lesser curve are very different lesions, and therefore the precision of the tests is necessary for proper diagnosis and treatment.

The Diaphragm

Here we integrate this major element of the deep fascial system, which, as a muscle, has a respiratory and ventilatory role: *respiratory*, because it is the vital motor of the pulmonary inspiration; *ventilatory*, because for the organism it is an important vector of visceral mobility and dynamic

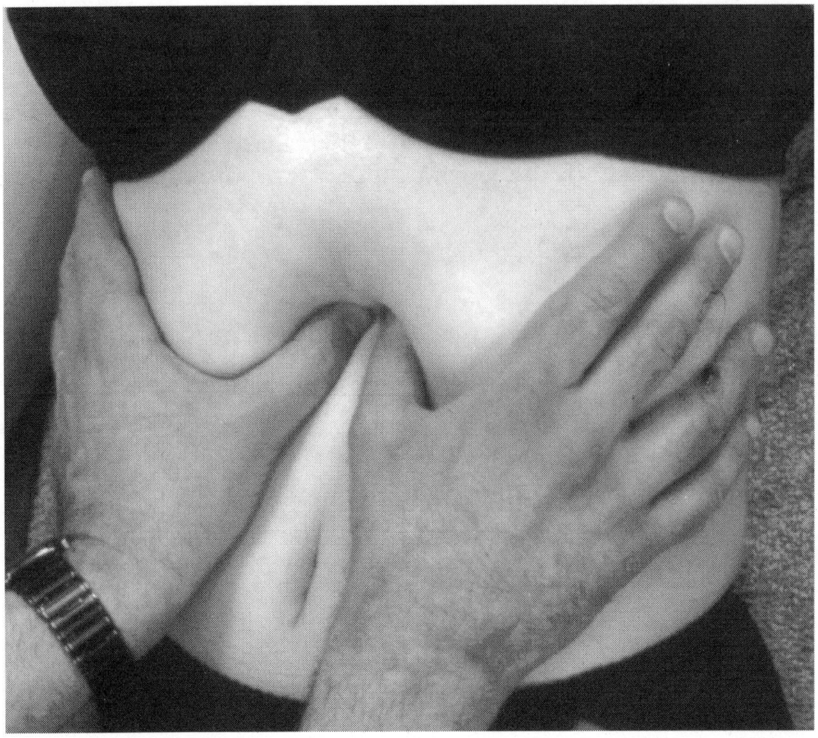

Figure 40

Test of the Central Tendon

circulation. The diaphragm in lesion may interfere with the passage of food into the stomach and therefore lead to digestive difficulty.

The most pertinent test that we have found is first to apply transverse traction on the phrenic center of the diaphragm, which is the aponeurotic center, the central tendon, and then to apply transverse traction on the muscular part of the diaphragm, on the right and on the left leaflets. We can also then test the right and left crura of the diaphragm.

Even if the diaphragm is rarely the site of a primary lesion, we must still give it a lot of consideration because treatment at this level may be critical for the complete osteopathic treatment. As A.T. Still wrote, the diaphragm must be taken into account in the search for the why of an illness.

The Gall Bladder

The particular sensitivity of this organ often causes it to react to the many stressful situations we may encounter in life. Osteopathic lesion of the gall bladder occurs in three stages:

- inflammation and spasm of the gall bladder;
- fibrosis and thickening of the muscular wall;
- gall stones.

The global test of the gall bladder is done underneath the costal margin at the 8th costal cartilage on the right, by pressing the organ into the (inferior) visceral border of the liver.

Even if the gall bladder has been removed, one should still test the tissular environment of the organ, where we will often find the residual imprint of fixations.

The Duodenum

The first part of the small intestine enfolds the head of the pancreas, which is deep inside the abdomen. Because this part of the digestive tract is firmly attached to the posterior wall, it is easy to locate by palpation. Using traction we test the following structures:

- the hepatoduodenal ligament, an important passage for the common bile duct, the portal vein, the hepatic artery, and of some lymphatic ganglions;
- the ligament of Treitz, from which the duodenojejunal junction suspends, and with which the crura of the diaphragm are connected;
- each portion of the duodenum, the most common lesion being the closure of the angle between D1 and D2.

The Jejunum and the Ileum

Being six meters long and very loosely fixated, the small intestine has a variable form and position. We test the root of the mesentery with the superior mesenteric artery and vein, which it contains, by longitudinally stretching the mesenteric root itself. We test the mesentery, from which are hanging the jejunum and the ileum, by using transverse traction. We then globally examine the mass of the small intestine by a series of pressure and traction tests centered around the umbilicus.

The Ileocecal Valve

This junction of the small intestine with the large intestine is the location of many osteopathic lesions, from the small muscular spasm of the valve to the pushing in of the ileum into the cecum.

We test this valve (and the ileocecal fold that lines it) in traction, so as to separate the ileum from the cecum.

The Vermiform Appendix

Usually located two centimeters below the ileocecal valve, its position varies, depending on the position of the cecum, which we should locate first. There are three reasons why the vermiform appendix merits serious attention:

- It is an organ proper to humankind and to all four-legged animals; a congenital absence is rare, suggesting that it has an important function.
- The vermiform appendix is located below the cecum, where all three colic taenia converge, and thus it represents the fascial link between these three longitudinal reinforcements of the large intestine.
- This organ is often inflamed and in spasm, and there are often adhesions following an appendectomy, so we often have to act upon this territory.

The vermiform appendix is the guardian of the ileocecal passage. It is hollow, and through it pass all liquids, which are analyzed. Infectious agents from outside, and under certain conditions the body's own biliopancreatic secretions themselves, may trigger an appendicular defensive reaction; causing the inflammatory or fibrotic state that we often find in this area. Subchronic appendicitis—both common and rarely suspected—is a tissular lesion easy to diagnose and treat using a Mechanical Link approach. (Acute appendicitis remains a purely surgical case).

Just because the appendix is difficult to locate does not mean that one should not try to locate, examine, and treat such an important structure. We test the vermiform appendix and especially its meso by applying inferior lateral traction.

The Large Intestine

We must test every portion of this last part of the digestive tube from the cecum to and including the rectum. For each portion we test the attachments, and, using longitudinal traction, we test the serous and muscular structure of the large intestine.

The lesions that we most often find on the large intestine are a fixation of the cecum, a closing of the right colic angle, and fixation at the root of the sigmoid mesocolon.

The Pelvic Girdle

We have already covered testing of the pelvis by lowering the ileum, opening the ileum, closing the ileum. The mechanism of these lesions and how to treat them is explained in the chapter on the ver-

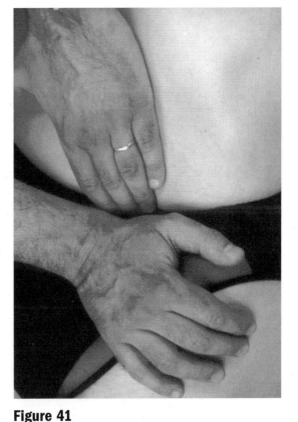

Figure 41

Test of the Sigmoid Mesocolon

Figure 42

Lowering Test of
the Ileum

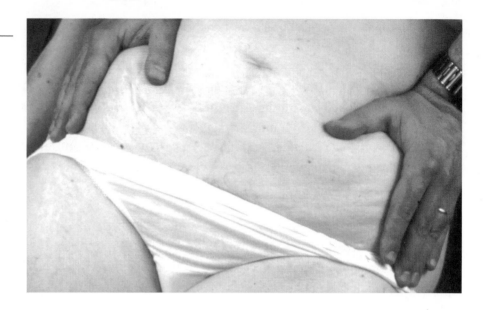

tebral functional unit. Many tests on the pelvis were done with the subject sitting up; in the following sections we add a few further tests that are more easily done with the patient supine.

The Inguinal Ligament

The frequency of the inguinal hernia in adults is evidence that there is a lot of tension in this region. The inguinal ligament forms the inferior border of the inguinal canal, through which, in males, run the ductus deferens and the testicular vessels. It also forms the superior border of the femoral arch, through which run the psoas muscle, the crural nerve, and the external iliac vessels. All fixations of the inguinal ligament will have an effect on the structures traveling through it.

We test it by applying longitudinal traction on the inguinal ligament from the ASIS to the pubic tubercule. We also bring the inguinal ligament inferior and superior.

The External Obturator Membrane

Lesions commonly develop here, and mostly relate to the coxofemoral articulation. We test by applying perpendicular pressure on the external surface of the membrane.

The Internal Obturator Membrane

Lesions here relate to the organs of the lower pelvis, and so we approach them via the abdomen. We test by applying perpendicular pressure on the internal surface of the membrane.

The Pelvic Diaphragm

This structure is part of the superficial fascial system. We can say that the pelvic diaphragm is a mirror image of the thoracic diaphragm with its phrenic center and domes. The pelvic diaphragm corresponds to the phrenic center, and the internal obturator membranes correspond to the right and left leaflets of the thoracic diaphragm. We test by applying pressure onto the pelvic diaphragm on the right and left side.

The Genital Sphere

The genital sphere is a highly sensitive territory that we must know how to approach without apprehension.

The Uterus

In Mechanical Link, we prefer to palpate externally—through the abdomen—rather than internally—through rectum or vagina—for many reasons:

- The proposed tests via the abdomen are precise and efficient; we have verified them all with endovaginal ultrasound and are confident that they act where they are supposed to.
- These tests are practical to apply; we are able to examine all patients easily, quickly, and without apprehension.
- These tests don't have the same contraindications as internal tests (infectious gynecological pathologies, menstruation, patient of minor age, moral, cultural, or religious restrictions, legal aspects, where the practitioner practices, etc.).

The tension tests that we do allow us to test the mechanical value of the connecting surface of the uterus in relation to its neighboring organs. The type of contact found here demonstrates the soft but resistant connection between the organs of the pelvis.

We should not be concerned with the normality of position of the uterus, but by mobilizing it in the possible spatial directions, we can evaluate the tissular flexibility of its fascial environment (functional diagnosis). These are the special directions we test:

- anterior and posterior uterus;
- right and left lateral uterus;
- right and left rotated uterus;
- superior traction of the uterus.

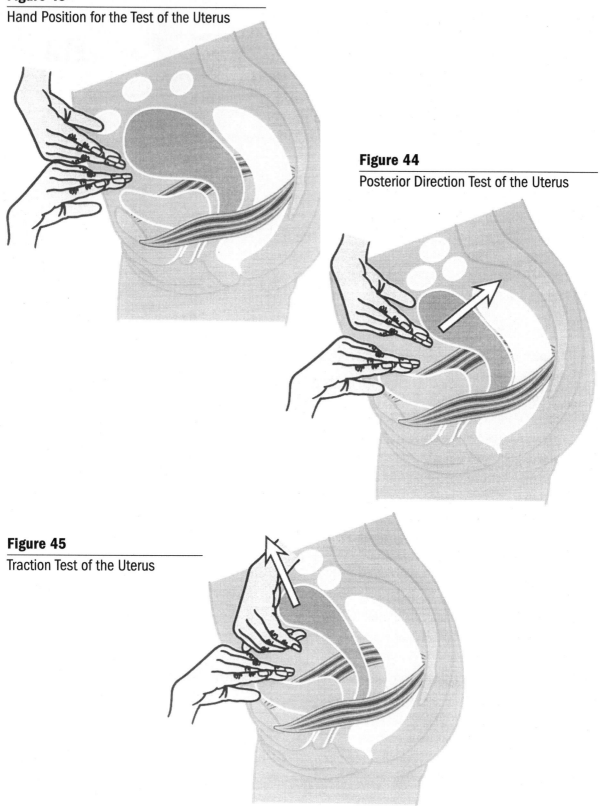

Figure 43

Hand Position for the Test of the Uterus

Figure 44

Posterior Direction Test of the Uterus

Figure 45

Traction Test of the Uterus

We also test the fallopian tubes and the right and left ovaries. The most common lesions are those of the left lateral uterus and the inferior position of the uterus.

The Prostate

Examination in the genital sphere will be reduced for men because the prostate has far fewer lesional possibilities than the uterus. We test this gland via the abdomen, applying tension to the right and left lateral prostate. The position of the prostate architecturally can be compared to that of the cervix in the uterus; in both places we find mostly the lesional fixation on the left.

We usually have good results with functional urinary trouble caused by a benign hypertrophy (adenoma) of the prostate.

The Urinary Tract

The Bladder

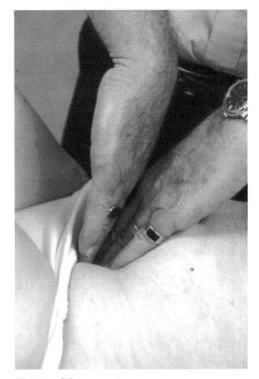

Figure 46
Posterior Movement Test of the Uterus

This musculomembranous organ is well anchored except at its superior surface, which is free and extensible so that the bladder's holding capacity can be increased. We first test the ligamentous attachments of the bladder, using traction:

- the anterior pubovesical ligament (which is also anterior puboprostatic in men);
- the lateral pubovesical ligaments which reach the lateral pelvic fascia on either side (lateral puboprostatic in men);
- the median umbilical ligament remains of the urachus continues above the umbilicus and becomes the round ligament of the liver.

We then test the vesicle dome by applying transverse traction, and the urethra by pulling the bladder superiorly.

Spasm or inflammation of the urethra, generally associated with an inferior fixation of the bladder, is often at fault in the functional urinary problems that osteopathy can often easily remedy.

The Kidneys

These are retroperitoneal organs that are very mobile because they are attached only to the diaphragmatic fascia. A kidney fixated in an inferior position is well known to the osteopath.

We test the kidneys by moving them superiorly or cephalically combined with rotation right and then rotation left.

We also test the ureters using longitudinal stretching, either globally, or in sections—high, middle, and low.

The Abdominal Organs

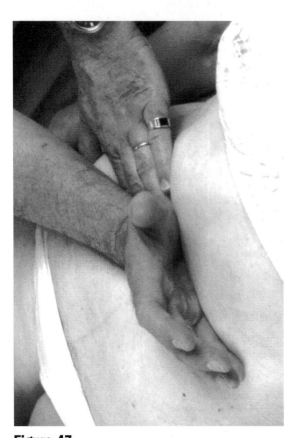

Figure 47

Test of the Head of the Pancreas

The Pancreas

This organ is so tight up against (and within the loop made by) the duodenum, that to access the head of the pancreas, one must also access the duodenum. The head of the pancreas must be tested in different ways:

•in relation to the second part of the duodenum, which we hold while stretching the pancreatic canal to the left and superiorly;

•in relation to the gall bladder, which we hold while stretching the common bile duct inferiorly.

Using traction we also test the body of the pancreas in relation to the transverse mesocolon, and more secondary, the tail of the pancreas in relation to the spleen.

The Spleen

Deeply buried in the left thorax, in its normal state, the spleen cannot be palpated. We test it using pressure, through the thoracic cage, at the level of the tenth rib. In practice, the specific or global tests of the spleen reveal little. It is the splenic artery that represents the real key to this organ, (covered in the chapter on the vascular system).

The Liver

This is the most voluminous organ of the body, and a fixation of the liver will greatly affect the mechanical balance of the abdomen and the general well-being of the organism. Even though global testing is useful, for greater precision we individually test each ligament of the liver and then the mobility of the organ around the three axes of rotation in space:

• falciform ligament;

- round ligament;
- coronary ligament;
- right and left triangular ligament;
- cephalic and caudal rotation around the coronary transverse axis;
- clockwise and counterclockwise rotation around the anteroposterior axis of the falciform ligament;
- right and left rotation around the vertical axis of the inferior vena cava.

It is common to have many restrictions of the liver, and the inhibitory balancing test will reveal the dominant lesion. The etiology of each fixation may be different. For example, a restriction of the coronary ligament is generally due to an emotional problem, such as frustration or repressed anger; whereas, a lesion of the falciform ligament tends to have a more metabolic origin, such as a hepatic overload. In any case, the normalization of a dominant lesion will always help the organism to adapt more effectively to the existing problem.

The Respiratory System

The tension tests that we recommend allow a detailed evaluation of the respiratory system, and osteopathic diagnosis here often corresponds to the clinical symptoms of the patient. We must not forget that inflammatory and infectious conditions often lead to osteopathic lesions that, if not treated, might lead to frequent recurrence or to chronic types of respiratory pathology.

The Larynx

This structure is at the same time a respiratory pathway and the principal speech organ.

We test the larynx by applying traction on its different cartilaginous parts. Fixation of the thyroid cartilage is the most common lesion.

The Trachea

Following the larynx, using traction we test the trachea, or airway, at the level of the cervical section, and then as it travels through the thoracic cage.

The Bronchial Tubes

Using traction we individually test the right and left primary bronchial tubes, from the bronchial bifurcation to the corresponding pulmonary hilum.

The Lungs

We do not so much test the lungs as the pleura and endothoracic fasciae that surround them. Fixations here will influence biomechanical ventilation, and therefore respiratory function. We test the mediastinum, which attaches at the hilum to form the pulmonary ligament. The test is done by fixating the anterior mediastinum and pushing the lung laterally. We also test the ligaments of the pleural dome, which suspend the pleura from the 7th cervical vertebra and intermittently from the 1st rib. We often find a lesion of the vertebropleural ligaments in pulmonary pathologies such as asthma, and it may also be a factor in lower cervical pain that radiates out to the upper extremities. The global test is done by applying caudal traction to the pleural dome. If necessary the specific test will allow us to localize which ligament is most serious.

The costal pleura will be tested globally by applying traction through the thoracic cage.

Fasciae Related to the Respiratory System

We examine fasciae related to the upper respiratory airways, such as the thyroid pocket and the connective capsule of the thymus:

- We test the mobility of the thyroid, as well as the global elasticity of the capsule that surrounds the right and left lobe, by elevating and

Figure 48

Pressure Test of the Left Pleural Dome (Global Test of the Suspensory Ligaments of the Pleural Dome)

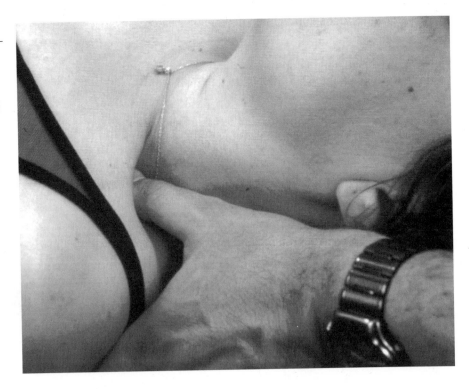

lowering it on the rail made by the trachea. Fixation of the thyroid inferiorly is common.

- We test the fascial capsule of the thymus by tractioning it inferiorly from the cervical fascia from which it is suspended. We mostly find lesion in this area in children, probably because the thymus remains a relatively voluminous and active lymphatic gland until puberty.

The Cardiac System

Just like all fascial and fibromuscular structures of the body, the heart responds well to the Mechanical Link approach. In our experience, manually releasing the different fixations that may affect this region will significantly improve cardiac function.

We test the heart by the intermediary of its surrounding fascia and with reference to its biomechanical context: in relation to the spine and the thoracic cage, as well as to the vascular system (covered in the next chapter).

The Bronchodiaphragmatic Membrane

This fibrous membrane that separates the anterior and the posterior mediastinum links the tracheal bifurcation above to the esophagus posteriorly, to the pericardium anteriorly, and to the diaphragm inferiorly. It acts as a reciprocal tension membrane that assures biomechanical cohesion between the different mediastinal organs. The fibers of this membrane are multidirectional; we test it by applying traction against the different organic structures to which it inserts.

We often find a lesion of this membrane in an anxious and reactive type of person who is often accompanied by much thoracic tightness, emotional dyspnea, and digestive problems. The release of this broncho-diaphragmatic membrane, if the lesion is dominant, will rapidly and permanently release many symptoms.

The Pericardium

We globally test the pericardium using a rocking action, by rolling the hand flat on its anterior topographic projection. If this global test reveals a dominant lesion, we will then specifically test each ligament:

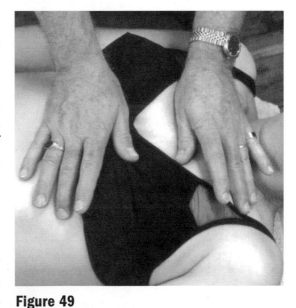

Figure 49

Traction Test of the Bronchodiaphragmatic Membrane

- superior sternopericardic ligament;
- inferior sternopericardic ligament;
- phrenicopericardic ligament;
- vertebropericardic ligament;

In this way we determine which element is responsible for the global fixation of the heart, which we can then adjust.

Quantity and Quality

The visceral unit is the one that requires the most tests for correct diagnosis. The different organic fixations are usually less significant (in relation to the total lesion) than those of the vertebral, thoracic, extremities, and cranial units. Thus, the visceral lesion is not often a primary lesion but mostly a dominant one that follows. The normalization of a visceral fixation in the position of the first or second dominant lesion is often the finishing touch on our treatment.

The practitioner that does not work in the visceral sphere cheats him or her self and the patients of an area of manual therapy that has marvelous results. In Mechanical Link, we insist on a complete evaluation of the visceral unit because we have noticed that intervention in this area will greatly refine our therapeutic action. If an adjustment on the knee or on an intraosseous line of force will efficiently mobilize a large quantity of energy, the visceral normalization will add subtleties to the treatment that are necessary for any quality approach to health.

12

The Vascular Unit

A History of the Heart

In evaluating the visceral system with specific tests of the structural fasciae of the organs (the meso, omentum, and ligament attachments, the fibrous, serous, and muscular sheaths), we know that these structures are not just attachments or protective coverings but also the medium through which the blood vessels and nerves travel to and from each organ. Although earlier in our work we had been quite satisfied with an approach that began and ended with attention to the fasciae, our work with the heart led us to adventures beyond the visceral ligamentous organization to the vascular system.

One day while carrying out our usual tension test, we found a heart fixed in an abdominal position (inferior). However, after further evaluation, we discovered that no ligamentous or diaphragmatic lesions maintained the heart in this lower position. We had to concede that something else was holding the heart in this position, and palpations revealed that increased tension in the abdominal aorta seemed to be responsible for this osteopathic lesion.

After lifting the lesion on the inferior heart using recoil, we then palpated the area and felt an increased elasticity and softness to the artery, using a test of longitudinal stretching. This confirmed our intuition: *large vessels such as the aorta may be the location of a tissular lesion of retraction*, and as a result, influence the mobility of the heart. Since then we have verified and confirmed the existence of this kind of lesion in thousands of patients.

Figure 50

Abdominal Fixation of
the Heart

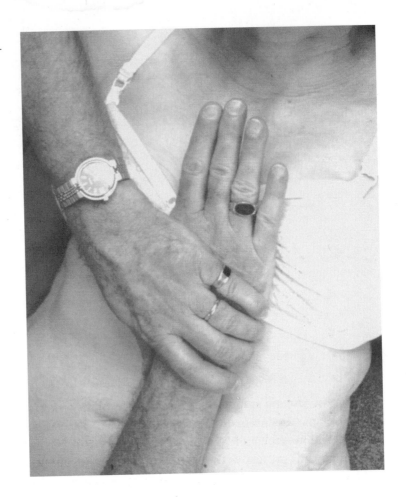

The heart is most often held in an inferior position by a restriction of
the abdominal aorta, but it may also be held in a superior position by an
exaggerated tension in the arch of the aorta and/or of its superior branches.
We must then differentiate between fixations of the *articular heart*, impli-
cating the pericardic ligaments, and lesions of the *vascular heart*, impli-
cating the larger vessels. These different osteopathic lesions need
differential tests.

The Osteopathic Lesion of the Artery

With this new perspective we started to systematically evaluate the vascular tree by testing all the arteries that we can access by palpation; they
are easy to locate, due to the pulse. By using the tension test, we simply,
but very delicately, without any compression, apply a longitudinal traction between two points that are located on the specific artery. We then

evaluate all the larger arterial branches, portion by portion, from the heart out to the extremities.

Like all other connective tissue, the internal, middle, and external layers of the artery are made up of elastic and collagen fibers as well as smooth muscular fibers. Large conductive arteries contain a greater proportion of elastic fibers, whereas medium sized arteries that distribute the blood contain a greater proportion of contractile fibers. In any case, this myofascial structure may be in osteopathic lesion: presenting a tissular restriction with all possible stages of inflammation and spasm, of fibrosis, or of sclerosis, stages we have already described. In doing a longitudinal traction test this fixation will be felt as a blockage, a clear resistance to stretching, whereas an artery should normally have a certain degree of elasticity and flexibility when under tension.

If we find many lesions in the vascular unit, we must use the inhibitory balancing test to find the most important lesion: the dominant lesion of the arterial system.

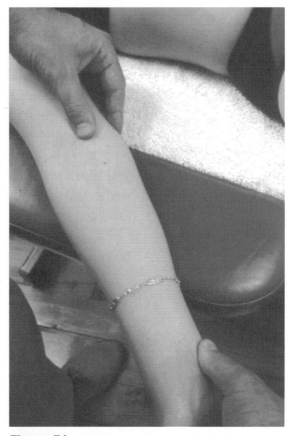

Figure 51

Tension Test of the Ulnar Artery

The Importance of the Artery in the Osteopathic Concept

When Still talked about the role of the artery, insisting on its preeminence, evidently he considered that he was stating a fundamental principle of osteopathy. At this time we can ask ourselves if that message was well understood; most manual practitioners nowadays limit their treatments to the articular structures only, thinking that by this means they will also adequately release any related vessels. Moreover, when an osteopath pays attention to the vascular system, it is generally only to look at lymphatic or venous return and carry out a few pumping or other maneuvers of drainage for relief of local symptoms.

The artery has become a "poor relation" in the modern osteopathic model, and so we were surprised by the results obtained by direct work at this level. The results have encouraged us to continue to explore an area that may turn out to be very important, even crucial.

The Biomechanical Role of the Artery

Though physiological knowledge of the dynamic exchanges performed by the artery is considerable, understanding of its biomechanical role remains minimal. To rectify this, we have studied the subject in detail, taking note of anatomy and any other clinical observations during our daily practice.

It must be noted that the arteries are located on the flexion side of an articulation. This strategic and privileged position prevents any excessive stretching during extension. In addition, due to the adipose tissue that surrounds and protects them, during extreme flexion there will be no abnormal compression. Since the artery is a vital structure for the organism, all mechanical functions seem to "articulate" around the vascular axis, so that it does not suffer any undue stress. *The artery is therefore an essential element that conditions the articular mechanism itself.*

Osteopathically we have noticed that a fixation of an artery always limits the mobility of the corresponding articulation: passively, by its own tension, and actively, by a defensive reflex that adds tension. The artery behaves like an *active ligament* (which it is anatomically at times, for example, the suspensory ligament of the ovary). Thus, one can observe that a fixation of a vertebral artery considerably limits cervical side-bending to the opposite side; fixation of the femoral artery limits the extension of the

Figure 52

Tension Test of the Left
Vertebral Artery

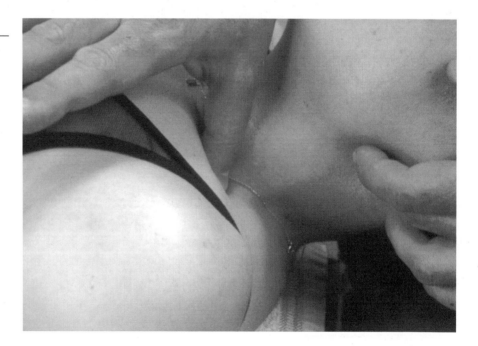

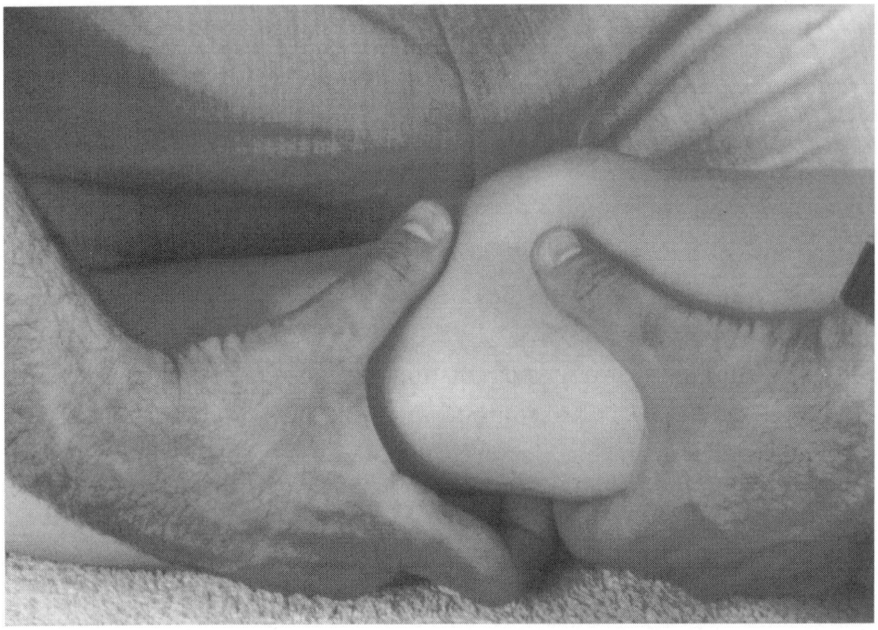

Figure 53
Tension Test of the Right
Popliteal Artery

elbow; one of the plantar artery limits the dorsiflexion of the ankle; etc.

With time, the restriction in an artery may lead to contractures:

- The classical reversal of the cervical curvature that remains after a motor vehicle accident is often due to a lesion in the common carotid artery combined with a lesion of the opposite vertebral artery.
- A flexion contracture of the hip may be associated with a lesion of the femoral artery.
- A flexion contracture of the knee is often maintained by fixation of the popliteal artery.

We can confirm this hypothesis by means of an osteopathic demonstration: the liberation of a vascular lesion by recoil will immediately restore mobility at the local articular system, sometimes in spectacular ways. If a heart held in an abdominal position is restored to a more superior position, the patient will regain ten to twenty degrees of thoracic extension. If the external iliac artery is released, the patient will regain the opposite lumbar side-bending, and so on, for all the lesions we have talked about.

We should not consider the artery as just a passive tube that carries the blood but also as an *active structure* that participates in the biomechanics of the body's organization. As such, it must be considered in the global osteopathic approach.

The Arterial System and the Venous System

From an osteopathic point of view, the artery is the master of the vascular system: *the artery governs the vein.* We observe that the venous system follows the arterial pathways. In conjunction with muscular contraction and thoracic ventilation this arterial-venous coupling constitutes the physiological motor of return circulation. The close relationship between artery and vein allows us to test both of them during our evaluation and specific treatment in the Mechanical Link approach. By targeting the arteries during tests and treatments (if necessary), we can address the entire circulatory system.

The Arterial System and the Muscular System

The metabolism of muscle tissue is highly dependent on its vascularization. A muscular contraction requires a lot of energy and at the beginning of the process only a small quantity of ATP (adenosine triphosphate, the major energy-carrying compound in cells) is available in the myofibers. During continuous activity the energy is supplied by the lactic acid glycogen process (anaerobic) and when sustained beyond thirty seconds, a biologic oxidation process (aerobic) that requires oxygen intake takes over.

The blood must therefore carry enough oxygen, glucose, and other nutrients (fatty acids, amino acids, and so on) to allow normal function. Many pathologies, from a simple case of muscle cramping to the infarcts of the myocardium, may be due to or predisposed by a deficiency in the vascularization.

At the functional level, we have noticed that a lesion of an artery is often associated with hypertonus of the corresponding muscle group. This hypertonicity will immediately be released once the restriction on the artery has been released. This relaxation of the muscle following the recoil performed on an artery might suggest to the osteopath that the muscular spasm itself is rarely primary, even though it is a factor in the lesional scheme of the concerned osteoarticular system. By addressing the vascular system we gain an original and efficient approach to stubborn and recurrent muscular problems (strains, cramps, tendonitis).

The Arterial System and
the Peripheral Nervous System

Just as the veins accompany the arteries, the nerves often use the same pathways. This anatomical structure is not random but due to the functional necessity of the organism. Because of it, all osteopathic work on the arteries will also have an effect on the vasculonervous package that accompanies it.

The neuron and its extension, the axon, are of ectodermic origin. The layer surrounding the nerve is of mesodermic origin, the same structure that surrounds the arteries and all other fasciae. In practice, we have noticed that fixations of the arteries follow the same pathways as conditions of neuralgia. For instance, the subclavian or brachial artery will have lesions in a case of cervicobrachial neuralgia, and the same is true for the external iliac artery in cruralgia or the popliteal artery for sciatica. In proof, we have demonstrated that specific adjustment on the artery in lesion will usually immediately release the pain of the corresponding neuralgia.

We believe that it may be interesting to look at the peripheral nerves in the same way that we have done with those related to the vascular tree, but at this point in our research we will continue to focus on the arteries that seem to be the key to the vasculonervous system.

The Arterial System and
the Autonomic Nervous System

The ability of the arteries to contract depends greatly on the sympathetic nervous system that accompanies the vessels and modulates the blood flow to meet the local and general needs of the organism. With trauma, the sympathetic system generates a reflexive vasoconstriction, and if this arterial spasm persists, constitutes the first stage of osteopathic lesion.

Each time that we do our traction test on a particular artery, we also stretch the sympathetic nervous filum that accompanies it. Acting in this manner on the arterial tunic and on the sympathetic system that accompanies it at the same time, represents Mechanical Link's original approach, offering practitioners a new access to the autonomic nervous system. This access is more direct than the classical access via the vertebrae that we already know.

Through osteopathic treatment of the arteries (and of the autonomic nervous system that accompanies them), we have the key to defuse the lesional mechanisms of certain pathologies in which the neurovascular origin is known, such as cramps, parasthesia, Raynaud's syndrome, neurodystrophy, functional arterial hypertension, etc.

The "Vascular Organs"

We have seen that we must differentiate between the articular heart and the vascular heart as being the site of two different types of fixations.

Myocardium originates embryologically from the mesoderm and from the beginning is part of the vascular fascial system. Two other organs have the same embryological parent: the kidneys and the spleen. (All others come from the endodermic layer from which develops the visceral system.) These three organs (heart, kidneys, and spleen) must be considered as having the same nature as the vascular system and so we must pay greater attention to the arteries on which they depend.

Physiologically the kidneys and the spleen are directly implicated in the functioning of the vascular system: the kidneys because they filter the blood, control the volume of blood circulating, and regulate arterial tension; the spleen because it holds a reserve of available blood, participates in the formation of lymphocytes, produces hemoglobin, and destroys red blood cells that are at the end of their usefulness.

Also without any doubt, the elements that make up the blood originate from the mesoderm; therefore, the blood itself is a *liquid fascial tissue*.

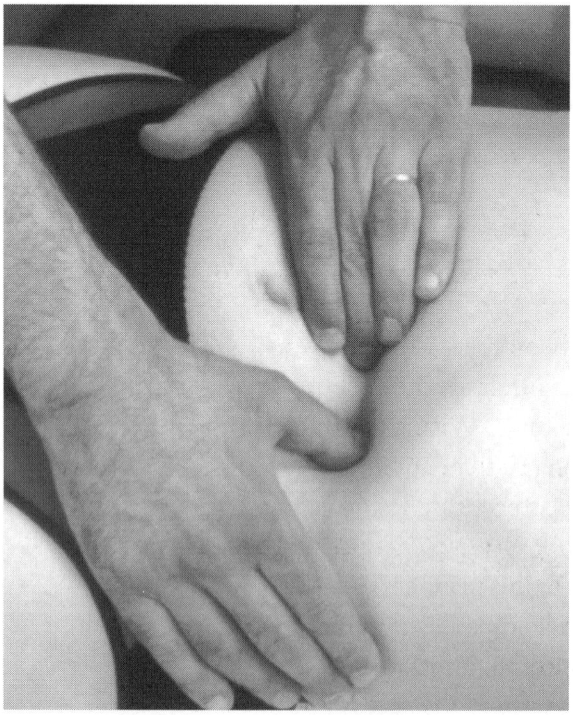

Figure 54

Tension Test of the Left Renal Artery

The Renal Artery

We consider the classical fixations of the kidneys when we systematically analyze them during our visceral evaluation. However, specific testing of the renal artery may uncover a lesion of the artery without there being a lesion of the organ itself. That is why, just as with the heart, it is so important to distinguish the *articular lesions* of the kidney—i.e. the restrictions of mobility in relation to its surroundings—from the *vascular lesions* of the kidney, which involve the artery itself but also affect the biomechanical and metabolic function of the organ. Note here that the kidney is hanging from the artery, and that the artery is an important attachment of the organ.

The Spleen Enigma

The spleen often poses a problem for the osteopath. We know the importance of its physiological functions, and Chinese medicine gives it a central place in the energetic regulation of the organism. The spleen is often implicated in traumas, especially car accidents, and our colleagues J.P. Barral and A. Croibier have written extensively on the subject.

We have so many reasons to be interested in this remarkable organ. The pressure test through the thoracic cage or the specific tests of all the ligamentous attachments or the mobilization of the spleen within its own loggia seem to tell us little and are rarely positive.

In Mechanical Link's approach we have solved the problem of testing by not only testing the spleen and its surrounding fascia, but more directly and particularly testing the splenic artery at the end of which it is suspended.

In practice, the spleen behaves like a vascular structure: i.e. fixation of the splenic artery is as common as fixation of the organ itself is rare. And just to show the functional dominance of the artery over the organ, study of anatomy reminds us that it is relatively common to find a multitude of small spleens along the splenic artery. This occurs in fifteen to thirty percent of all people, as though the spleen or spleens were in actuality only an extra growth of the vascular axis. This might also explain why the removal of the spleen seems to have little medical consequence. Thus, we should consider the organ but give even more importance to the vascular system to which it is connected and upon which it functionally depends. It is important to know how to test and treat the splenic artery, which is the key to biochemical function of the spleen.

The Arterial Lesion and Traumatic Sequelae

The examination of the vascular system must be integrated with that of all other functional units; we focus on it in isolation only when we treat local symptoms in emergency cases. In an acute sprain, for example, the vascular troubles appear rapidly, and letting them remain untreated will interfere with the natural process of healing. In the same way homeopathy uses arnica in cases of trauma, (and it is mostly a vascular remedy), we must quickly intervene in the circulatory disturbances connected with trauma. In emergency cases we systematically treat by locally targeting the joint involved and then the local vascularization in order to immediately release the vascular lesions that are taking place.

It is often surprising to see how a simple adjustment on an arterial lesion will immediately decrease swelling and hematoma that may have been there for some time. In our clinic we have also demonstrated that pain will also decrease, either right away or very shortly after the normalization of an arterial lesion. The functional recuperation seems to be quicker and more complete if we treat the vascular component of the lesional chain. Thus, we think that the systematic integration of the vascular system (like the integration of the lines of force) is a key element in emergency treatments.

Osteopathy and Prevention of Vascular Alterations

Aging that leads to hardening of the arteries is an ineluctable process. We are all aware of the high incidence of cardiovascular pathologies causing death, and so it is very important to develop approaches to prevention.

Osteopathic treatment of the arteries is a very efficient way to maintain flexibility and elasticity in the vascular system. The specific tension tests often allow us to detect an early stage of fixation in an artery, even in the absence of noticeable pathology. The recoil treatment allows a gentle normalization of this type of lesion. For long-term health management, osteopathy is a preventive approach of choice because taking care of our vascular structure allows us to slow down the aging of our arteries.

The Treatment

After evaluation comes treatment, during which we neutralize all of the arterial lesions. The adjustment must have the same criteria as the tension test: that it be precise, quick, efficient, pain free, and without contraindication.

The normalization of an arterial lesion is done by recoil. The concerned arterial segment is put under tension just as with the traction test, until the fascial barrier that characterizes all osteopathic lesions is reached. Then, we only have to go beyond the tissular barrier by quickly increasing the previous tension test. Just like all direct techniques, the recoil goes against the resistance; we aim—in a very minute way—to "stretch" the arterial portion beyond the fascial restriction.

The four phases of the recoil technique (as described in Chapter 6) may be performed on the arteries. The only particularity of the adjustment on an artery, due to the great sensitivity of this structure, is in the lightness and the fineness (subtlety) of the gesture: the recoil must be like a *puff of air*, as if we wanted to find the origin of the artery ("are" = air, "teveo" = carry).

The Sovereignty of the Artery

Work on the arteries needs much more precision than we are able to describe in this chapter. Our larger aim is not to be exhaustive or didactic but to invite reflection on the primary importance of the vascular system in the osteopathic approach. Following that fundamental principle, in our practice we seek to do several things:

- Be able to evaluate the whole arterial unit with ease and speed using the tension tests that we have presented here.
- Know how to objectively compare the osteopathic lesion of an artery to any fixation in other functional units diagnosed during the evaluation—made possible by the inhibitory balancing test.
- Be able to selectively adjust an arterial restriction—easily and efficiently done using the recoil technique.

In some cases an arterial lesion will be secondary and will not need treatment because it will normalize with the adjustment of the major restrictions in another system. In other cases, an arterial fixation may end up being a primary or dominant lesion, one that we must liberate in order to completely and permanently neutralize all other fixations that in the hierarchy depend on it.

We would like to dedicate this research to the one that has presented the fundamental principle of osteopathy, the one whose visionary intuition caused him to state that "the role of the artery is absolute."

13

The Cephalic Unit

Starting from *Cranial Osteopathy*

When W.G. Sutherland discovered fluctuation of the cerebrospinal fluid and with that knowledge developed a whole new manual approach to the craniosacral system, the Still osteopathic approach was expanded. Practitioners such as H.I. Magoun, V. Fryman, and J. Upledger transmitted their precious knowledge to practitioners, and the cranial approach is now an integral part of the therapeutic repertoire of all well-versed osteopaths.

It became clear to us that we could not neglect this approach to the cranium and, at the same time, it was difficult to integrate the listening techniques or the functional techniques into our usual Mechanical Link protocol. Several questions needed to be considered, and to answer each we looked for a concrete answers using our hands:

- Is a cranial osteopathic lesion fundamentally different than a vertebral, visceral, or peripheral articular one?
- How could the dominant lesion of the pathomechanical cranium be determined?
- How could we examine the cranium in a way similar to the methods used for other functional units, and therefore produce comparable results that could be integrated with the rest of the system?
- How could we handle atypical lesions of the cranium such as those related to the teeth, the sinuses, or the intraosseous lines of force?
- Should we start osteopathic treatment at the cranium or at a distance?
- Can we normalize a cranial osteopathic lesion with just the recoil?

Developing Mechanical Link
of the Cephalic Unit

Even in accepted professional usage the term *cranial* is not exact. Using the term may wrongly imply that there are different osteopathic specialties or that the cranium is so particular that it must be considered apart from other functional units. In fact, anatomically speaking the cranium is only the osseous box that contains the encephalon. That's why we prefer the term *osseous head* or *cephalic unit* so as to include the bones of the face and the mandible, which are also of importance.

The osseous head is divided into three parts: the *inferior floor*, composed of one mobile bone, the mandible; the *middle floor*, or the face, where the sensory organs are located; the *superior floor*, or the cranium, which contains the encephalon.

Functionally this cephalic unit is connected with all other biomechanical units of the body by the three great fascial systems: superficial, deep, and dura mater. All osteopathic lesions of the cephalic unit will influence the rest of the body, and vice versa; this makes it illusory to approach the cephalic unit independently from other parts of the body.

We examine the osseous head with the patient supine, by means of a series of preestablished tension tests in order to find all the lesions that are present. As for the other connective structures of the body, the tension tests are done by applying pressure or traction on the different key points of the cephalic skeleton. As always, an element of the osseous head will be considered in osteopathic lesion if, during the tension test, there is a clear and definite resistance: a blockage we can feel as a rigidity of the structure being tested. Unlike the osteopathic cranial listening technique, we directly provoke the structure by using a light but sufficient tension in order to obtain a clear indication of its degree of fixation.

Although the pressure and traction tension tests are sufficient for giving a precise and exact diagnosis of the lesional organization of the cephalic unit, those not yet familiar enough with the practice of Mechanic Link can verify results using the classical functional cranial test. It will be discovered that the results will be the same.

The tension tests that we have developed are done very quickly; we analyze the whole cephalic skeleton in a short period of time, i.e. sixty tests in less than two minutes. To be systematic, tests are done following a spiral shape, starting from the mandible and exploring all the key points of the osseous head, and these will guide us to the sphenobasilar symphysis.

Figure 55

Tension Test of the Osseous Head

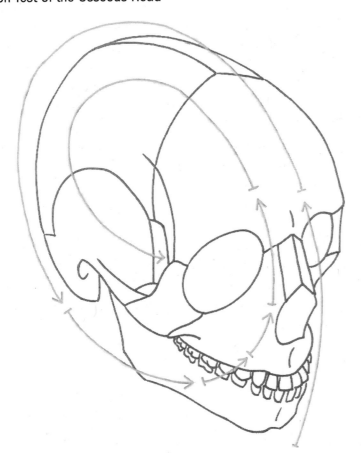

Diagnosis of the cephalic sphere concludes with the specific test of the ossification centers—the beam of the cranium and the intraosseous line of force of the facial skeleton—osseous structures that belong to the line of force functional unit but may be examined, for convenience, with the cephalic functional unit.

This protocol we have devised addresses the following areas, in the order given:

- the floors of the cephalic unit;
- the dura mater system;
- the temporomandibular module;
- the teeth;
- the maxillofacial skeleton;
- the cavities of the osseous head;
- the cranial sutures;
- the cranial bumps (ossification centers);
- the lines of force of the osseous head.

The Three Floors of the Cephalic Unit

The division of the head into three parts corresponds to embryological, anatomic, neurological, architectural, geometric, energetic, and symbolic realities.

Inferior Floor

This is a test of the symphysis mentae and a global test of the mandible. We test by applying anteroposterior pressure with the thumb while the patient is comfortably supine.

Middle Floor

This is a specific tension test of the intermaxillary suture and a global test of the facial skeleton.

We apply the same anteroposterior pressure, but this time on the point between the nose and the upper lip.

Figure 56

The Three Floors

The Three Floors	Embryology	Anatomy	Neurology	Architecture	Geometry	Energetic	Symbolic
Superior Floor	Frontonasal Protuberance (Neurocranium)	Cranium	Ophthalmic Nerve V–1	Vaults and Arches	The Circle: The Calvaria has the shape of a dome.	Cerebral Floor, Intellectual Functions	The World Above
Middle Floor	Maxillary Protuberance of the 1st Brachial Arch (Viscerocranium of the Face)	Osseous Face	Maxillary Nerve V–2	Pillars and Beams	The Triangle: The Maxilla has the shape of a triangular pyramid.	Rhythmic Floor, Sensorial Functions	The Intermediary World
Inferior Floor	Mandibular Protuberance of the 1st Brachial Arch (Viscerocranium of the Mandible)	Mandible	Mandibular Nerve V–3	Foundation and Crypt	The Square: The Mandible has the shape of a cube.	Metabolic Floor, Instinctive Functions	The World Below

Figure 57

The Three Floors of the Osseous Head

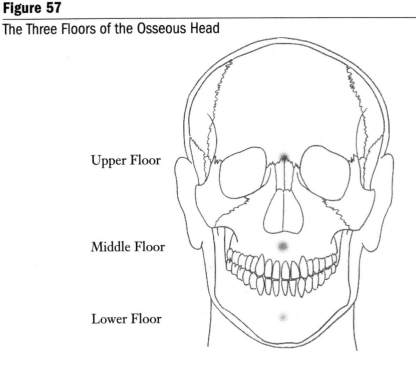

Upper Floor

Middle Floor

Lower Floor

Figure 58

The Dura Mater System

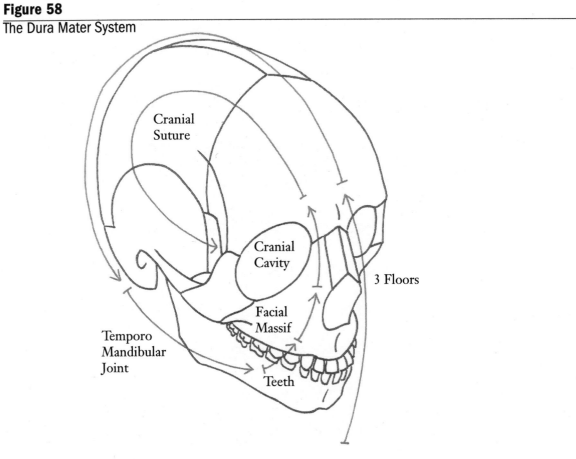

Cranial
Suture

Cranial
Cavity

3 Floors

Facial
Massif

Temporo
Mandibular
Joint

Teeth

Figure 59

The Three Floors in Detail

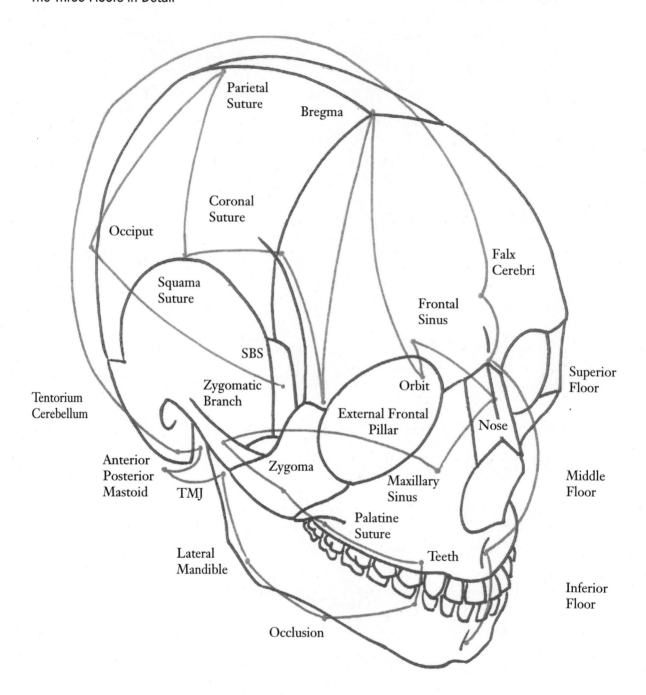

Parietal
Suture

Bregma

Coronal
Suture

Occiput

Falx
Cerebri

Squama
Suture

Frontal
Sinus

SBS

Zygomatic
Branch

Orbit

Superior
Floor

External Frontal
Pillar

Tentorium
Cerebellum

Nose

Anterior
Posterior
Mastoid

Zygoma

TMJ

Maxillary
Sinus

Middle
Floor

Palatine
Suture

Lateral
Mandible

Teeth

Inferior
Floor

Occlusion

Superior floor

This is a specific tension test of the nasofrontal suture and a global test of the cranial vault.

The test is done is the same manner, using anteroposterior pressure, but this time at the junction of the nasal and frontal bone. If no lesions are present, the practitioner's thumb will be able to sink in at each floor level.

At the beginning, we thought that these tests were enough to diagnose an osteopathic lesion of the osseous head that may have participated in the total lesion of the body. However, experience showed that the cephalic unit could not be satisfactorily approached using only those three tests; certain fixations may end up being primary or dominant without having that floor in lesion. We then developed more tests for the evaluation of the osseous head, as follows.

Figure 60

Global Test of the Cranial Vault

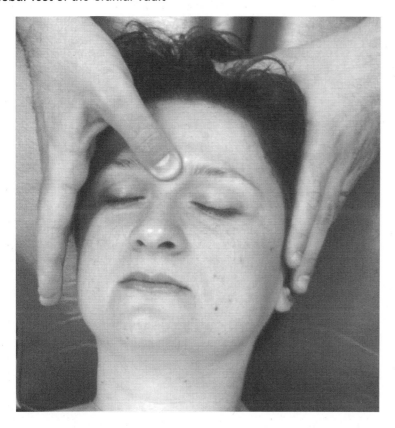

The Dura Mater System

The dura mater or external meninges, is a connective tissue of mesodermic origin (differing from the pia mater and the arachnoid that originates from the ectoderm just as does the nervous system that it surrounds). Since a fascial structure is susceptible to osteopathic lesions, we need to include in the general evaluation of the cephalic unit the cranial dura mater, as well as its different expansions such as the falx cerebri, the falx cerebelli, the tentorium cerebellum, and the spinal dura mater that links the occiput to the sacrum. We test by applying traction.

The membranes of reciprocal tension of the cranium are the same as an architectural support that prevents the spreading of the walls or the rope between the legs of a double ladder that stabilizes it. An abnormal fixation on the dura mater will influence the flexibility of the bones to which it attaches.

Figure 61

Test of the Falx Cerebri

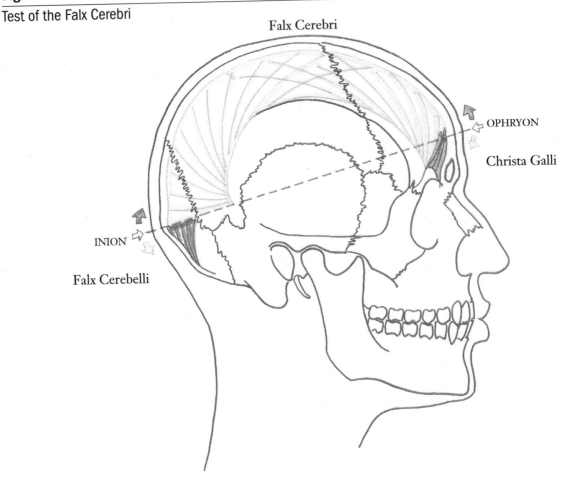

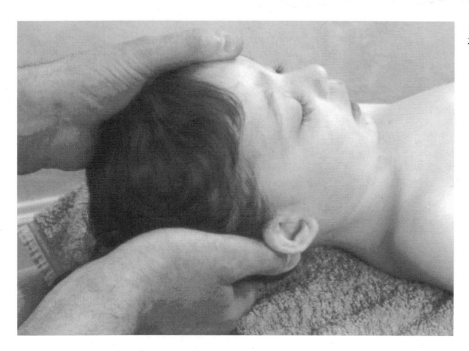

Figure 62
Test of the Falx Cerebri

The Temporomandibular Module

We don't need to go into detail about the mechanics of the temporo-mandibular module because many books have been written on the subject. To approach the temporomandibular module several tests are necessary:

The Anterior and Posterior Test of the Mastoid Process

The mastoid process is an osseous piece of the temporal bone that originates from the auditory capsules of the cartilaginous neurocranium (as distinguished from the squama of the temporal that originates from the membranous neurocranium). It needs a specific test. The mastoid forms one of the four principal pillars of the cranial building, and is therefore submitted to great stress. Most often a bilateral fixation of the mastoids features one mastoid rotated anterior and one rotated posterior. (We also find this kind of "torsion" in the clavicles and the ilium).

Lateral Translation Test of the Mandible

This test involves lateral gliding, which differs from the natural deduction movement, and cannot be created voluntarily by the subject. A right or left lateral fixation of the mandibular angle is often related to a nonverbal emotional state.

Figure 63

Global Test of the
Temporomandibular
Articulation

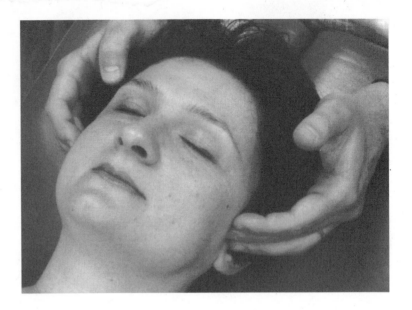

The Compression Test of the Mandible

This global test, involves compressing the mandibular condyle into the temporal socket, and when positive, is a sign of an imbalance in the dental occlusion. If this malocclusion ends up being the primary or dominant lesion, we must analyze the intraosseous line of force of the mandible and the intraosseous line of force of each tooth.

The Temporomandibular Articulation Test

Being the only articulation of the cephalic unit that is really mobile, it requires a global test to see if there is a restriction. In that case, many specific tests will be needed to determine on which parameters the adjustment will take place.

The Teeth

Although the teeth are mostly used to chew food and so belong to the digestive system, we prefer to approach the teeth within the anatomical context of the osseous head. As we have seen in the chapter on embryology, except for the enamel that covers the crown, the teeth are mesodermic tissue, like the osteoarticular system of the body with which it is integrated. To describe the topography of the teeth, we use the standard international nomenclature.

In osteopathy, we must recognize the importance of the teeth and some of the things that can affect them: lesional sequelae due to direct shock, the effect of dental care or orthodontic apparatus, occlusion imbalance, infections, and so on. Many energetic dental practitioners have established a relationship between the teeth and our general health, and especially the relationship between them and the organs in our body's somatotopies or the function of the meridians that pass through them. Our osteopathic approach is to act on the tooth that is the most fixated during our tension test, and not on any showing local symptoms or possible distant effects.

During examination of the osseous head, we first systematically test by applying global pressure in the four dental quadrants. We can consider each quadrant and the teeth in that area as a unit, and if there is a restriction in that quadrant, each tooth will be individually tested to find out which one is at fault. Because we test the alveolar cavity of teeth, we can test each the same way, whether it is a healthy tooth, one with an apparatus, a prosthesis, or even the site of an extracted tooth (by testing the osseous scar). For many reasons the canine is a special tooth. Since its root is the deepest in the bone, it forms the main pillar of the maxillomandibular architecture. It is statistically the one that is most often in lesion.

The recoil, due to the extreme precision of its impact, allows us to easily adjust all the different parameters of fixation of a tooth in lesion.

The Maxillofacial Skeleton

There are usually many osteopathic lesions in the bones of the face; the face remains very exposed to aggressions. To be able to properly evaluate the biomechanics of the face, many tests are needed.

The Suture of the Hard Palate

We have established two tests to evaluate the median suture and the transverse suture without having to test internally.

The Zygoma

The cheekbones are the victims of numerous shocks. We must test the zygoma by global decompaction, and then if necessary test each possible area of restriction.

The Zygomatic Process of the Temporal Bone

The osseous process is a lever for the rotation of the squama of the temporal and a true flying buttress for the cephalic building. This double function, mechanical and architectural, calls for two different tests: a mobility test carried out by lowering and elevating, a "cranking" of the anterior and posterior rotation of the squama of the temporal; an intraosseous test to feel the flexibility of the flying buttress.

The Base of the Mastoid

This osseous structure, built on the mastoid pillar like a marquee, gives rise to the lateral arch of the cranium that is linked to the zygomatic pillar (superior temporal line). It is also an important attachment for the superficial cervical aponeurosis. To test the base of the mastoid we only have to apply pressure on the bone just posterior to the ear.

The Cavities of the Osseous Head

The principal cavities of the cephalic skeleton are the nasal fossa, the paranasal sinus, and the orbits.

The Nasal Fossa

These are the beginning of the superior airways and the location of olfaction. We must perform two specific tests:
- The nasal septum (osseous and cartilaginous) by applying perpendicular pressure at the bridge of the nose. This test acts directly on the ethmoid sinus.
- The lateral walls of the nasal walls by applying pressure on each side, on the nasal bone, and on the ascending branch of the maxilla.

These are often the site of traumatic sequelae and/or surgeries.

The Paranasal Sinuses

These cavities have the same architectural function (reinforcing the osseous wall) as the galleries above the aisles in a church that increase the resistance of the lateral walls. We must individually test each maxillary and frontal sinus; the ethmoid sinus is tested during the previous test of the nasal septum.

A surprising number of fixations are found on the sinuses, and they are also the location of many infections, chronic or acute, that lead to tissular inflammation and then progress to osteopathic lesions. With the specific approach of the Mechanical Link, we often have good results with recurring pathologies such as rhinitis and sinusitis, either in acute cases by symptomatic targeting treatment of that territory, or in chronic cases by the treatment of the total osteopathic lesion.

The Orbit

We test the cavity of the eye by distracting the frontal bone from the zygoma, maxillary, sphenoid, and nasal bones so that the orbital cavity is opened superiorly; a fixation at this level generally leads to a palpable hypertension of the eyeball (functional hypertension because it reverses immediately following a correction of the orbital opening by means of the recoil technique).

The Cranial Sutures

We agree with those who insist that the cranium *moves*. We test each principal suture of the cranial vault, even if fixations of these areas are not as common as might be thought. The possible micro movements at this level and the direction of the pressure or traction for the tests depend on the anatomy of each concerned suture.

We give a lot of importance to two precise points of the cranial dome that we systematically test:

- bregma, the junction of the coronal and sagittal sutures, is the true keystone of the calvaria because this point corresponds to the anterior fontanel, the last presutural junction to close;

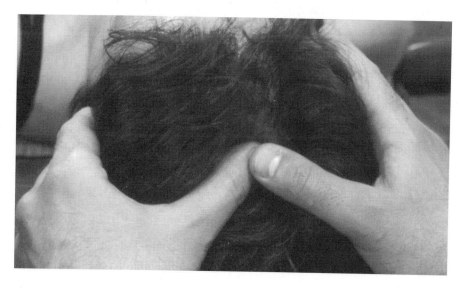

Figure 64

Pressure Test of Bregma

Figure 65

Traction Test of the
Temporoparietal Suture

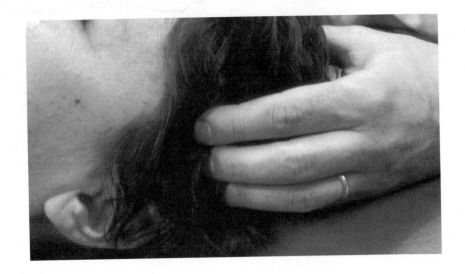

- lambda, junction of the sagittal and lambdoid sutures, is the second keystone of the cranium (posterior fontanel).

The fixation of these points always has a great influence on people's general health, and we have had spectacular results by releasing bregma or lambda.

We finish the evaluation of the cranial sutures with a global test of the sphenobasilar symphysis. If this test is positive, we must then obtain more detail by analyzing the different movements of the sphenoid in relation to the occiput:

- flexion and extension;
- right and left rotation;
- right and left side-bending;
- right and left lateral translation (strain);
- superior and inferior vertical strain;
- decompaction;
- diastasis.

The correction of the lesion must be done on the lesion of most severe restriction that was found during the specific evaluation.

The Cranial Ossification Centers

These protuberances of the frontal, parietal, and occipital bones represent the primary ossification centers of the fetal cranium. The intraosseous lesion of these cranial bumps will be felt as a point resistant to pressure.

The Occipital Ossification Center

This place corresponds with the instinct function of an individual, and a fixation at this level is often found in the newborn. The spot relates to the oral phase of Freudian psychoanalysis.

The Parietal Ossification Center

This place relates to the emotional system, and lesions here are mostly found in children and women. The spot corresponds with the anal phase of psychoanalysis.

The Frontal Ossification Center

This area relates to the mental function, and a blockage here is quite common in adults. It corresponds to the Oedipus complex of psychoanalysis.

For all the cranial ossification centers, the right side indicates a recent problem; the left one more ancient or a deeper trouble of the personality. The adjustment of a cranial ossification center often brings about a significant release of a neurotic state (for instance, anxiety, or depression) that the patient may suffer.

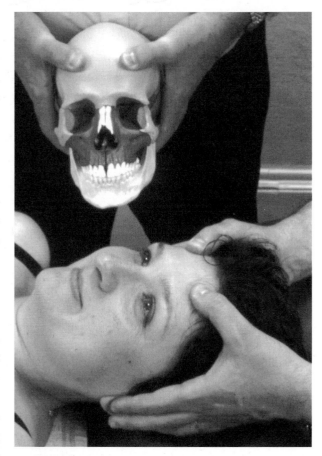

Figure 66
Pressure Test of the Two Frontal Ossification Centers

The Intraosseous Lines of Force of the Cephalic Unit

These can be examined while diagnosing the amount of restriction in the cephalic unit or when examining the intraosseous lines of force functional unit. The test of a line of force is done by longitudinal compression of the involved osseous segment, either with two fingers doing the test or with one finger and a counter force at the other end. The sign of a lesion in an intraosseous line of force is that it is impossible to compress the segment.

For the cephalic unit we must systematically evaluate these intraosseous lines of force:

- the beams at the base of the cranium—the sphenofrontal beam and the petrous beam that converge on an oblique axis on the sella turcica;
- the pillars of the cranium—the frontal pillar, the zygomatic pillar, the mastoid pillar, and the occipital pillar;
- the pillars of the face—the pillar of the chin, the mandibular pillar, the canine pillar, the nasal pillar;
- the zygomatic arch (flying buttress), that links the zygomatic and the mastoid pillar;
- the dental area;

Not only are lesions of the intraosseous line of force extremely common, but this kind of lesion is often primary or dominant, and so, necessary to treat.

Treatment Protocol

In our treatment we give the same amount of emphasis to the cephalic unit that we give to other functional units. By doing the inhibitory balance test we find out which is the dominant lesion of the cephalic unit, and then do an inhibitory balancing test with all the other seven functional units—vertebral, thoracic, visceral, etc.—to find the primary lesion.

The first adjustment will always be on the primary lesion that we have found with the inhibitory balancing test. If the primary lesion is in the cephalic unit, we correct it by means of the recoil technique, following the protocol that we have already presented. The recoil is easily applied and always performed the same way, no matter which structure is implicated (the tension membrane, the temporomandibular articulation, a tooth, a sinus, a cranial suture, etc.).

If the primary lesion is located elsewhere, on another functional unit, of course that is where the treatment has to start. After that we verify the effect of that adjustment on the lesions of the cephalic unit. If they were secondary they will have been released without having to work on them.

Whether the corrections are local or at a distance, the normalization effect on the cephalic unit will be felt immediately, which can be verified by palpation of the cranial sphere (postural behavior of the cranium) or by a classical listening test involving the cranial rhythm. In the Mechanical Link approach, treating the osseous head, or cephalic unit, requires working with it as part of the total lesion and intervening only *where it is needed, when it is needed, and how it is needed.*

14
The Dermis Unit

The Cutaneous Lesion

The integument that covers the outer layer of the body is the skin (epidermis, dermis, and hypodermis) and its annexes (hair, sebaceous and sudoriparous glands, nails). The epidermis and its annexes develop from the ectoderm (just as the nervous system does), whereas the dermis, the hypodermis, and the superficialis fasciae originate from the mesodermic layer. Thus, the dermis is a type of connective tissue; it will react the same as the osteoarticular system and the visceral system to our osteopathic approach.

Positive results from treatment of the dermis stimulated us to integrate the integument into Mechanical Link as its own functional unit, at the same level as the vertebral column, the visceral unit, or the osseous head.

The integument system can be considered as an organ, and it has many functions:
- thermal and mechanical protection of the body;
- sensory perception;
- elimination through sweat;
- synthesis of vitamin D;
- protection (immune barrier)
- etc.

In traditional Chinese medicine (TCM), the skin is associated with the lung (respiration) and the large intestine (elimination) as well as with the circulation of defensive energy (the immune system). So, the skin is

Figure 67

Cleavage Lines of the Dermis

From Benninghof

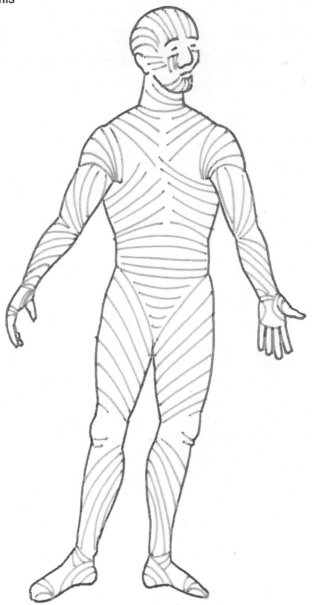

not just an inert cover but is an important vital structure that we must integrate into our osteopathic treatment.

The dermalgia (skin pain) described by Jarricot in his seminars, the connective reflexive zones of R. Peronneaud Ferre, and the cutaneous somite segments of G. Gesret all point to the therapeutic and diagnostic importance of work at this level. Thus, we knew we had to approach the skin as a functional unit and be able to compare a fixation of the dermis with other osteopathic lesions (through the inhibitory balancing test) in order to determine the primary lesion. The following is Mechanical Link's unique approach to the cutaneous tissue.

Like other connective tissue, the dermis, or chorion, is made of collagen and elastic fibers that adhere to one another and are oriented following certain tension lines. (This organization of the dermic network reminds us of the intraosseous line of force). We have noticed that the longitudinal routes of these cleavage lines follow the dermatomes. Observation of healing after surgery tells us that a cut parallel to these cutaneous lines makes for less severe scarring, whereas a perpendicular cut breaks the collagen spindles and leads to a thicker scar. In the same way, excessive tension of the dermis during pregnancy or during too rapid growth will create a transverse tear of these lines and lead to the unsightly stretch mark that many women complain about.

Scars as Fixations

If we have described an osteopathic lesion in general as being a fascial scar, we can consider that a scar of the skin is a particular case of an osteopathic fixation.

The study of the cutaneous movement to reestablish homeostasis perfectly illustrates the scarring process. The healing of an assault on the epidermis layer only (of ectoderm origin) is brought about by a renewing of the cells, which allows a reestablishment of the integrity of this superficial level of the cutaneous layer. The scarring of the dermis, similar to the scarring of all tissues that originate from the mesoderm, will follow a more complex route schematized in three steps:

- *The inflammatory phase:* vasodilatation, formation of blood clots, and the arrival of white blood cells that will engulf and digest the microbes. The cells of the dermis will transform into fibroblasts that will synthesize the collagen fibers.
- *The fibrosis phase,* called the "productive phase": formation of the neo-collagenic tissue, in which the density of the fibers is already greater than those of the normal cutaneous tissue. The orientation of the fibers is parallel to the longitudinal axis of the scar.
- *The sclerosis phase:* pathological hardening of the scarring connective tissues that are lacking in all vascularization. This will give a keloid scar of more or less hypertrophied and adherent appearance.

No matter what kind of the attack on the cutaneous area (trauma, burn, surgery) many practitioners in alternative medicine consider a badly healed scar the source of mechanical and energetic disturbances. Certainly, the hardening or retraction of the scarring tissue creates a nociceptive stimulation of the local cutaneous receptors (especially the ones that are very sensitive to the stretching of Ruffini's corpuscles and Meissner's corpuscles) that may then generate a reflexive postural imbalance on one or more corresponding dermatomes and become the determining element in an osteopathic lesional chain.

Protocol

Our goal must be to integrate the dermis, and especially the cutaneous scars, during our Mechanical Link evaluation. In practice, to be able to test the elasticity of the dermis, we must put the skin under tension by placing our hand flat on an area and applying a gentle traction along the longitudinal axis of the cleavage lines of the skin. (That trajectory has been well described by Benninghof. See Figure 67.) This traction on the collagen fibers of the dermis also glides the layer on top along the one below, and this plane of gliding is at the level of the fatty layer of the hypodermis that forms the junction between the dermis and the superficialis fasciae. (Or, when the latter is not present, to the superficial fasciae.)

The hypodermis carries the vessels and the nerves of the skin, and we must note the importance of the cutaneous tissue as a blood reservoir, a vascular reserve that represents close to ten percent of the blood volume of the body. (Note once again, how the mechanical vascular and neurological links are closely associated, if not indivisible.)

When there is a fixation, the hand feels a clear resistance at the point of traction or gliding. We will then consider this fascial barrier as part of the total lesion, and so it will be balanced against the other fixations found during the general evaluation. In all cases, a lesion of the dermis can be verified by a skin roll that will clearly and objectively show an abnormally thick and more sensitive area.

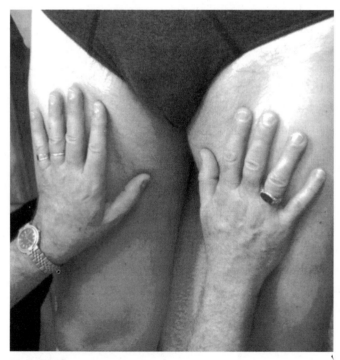

Figure 68

Gliding Test of the Dermis at the Level of the Thighs

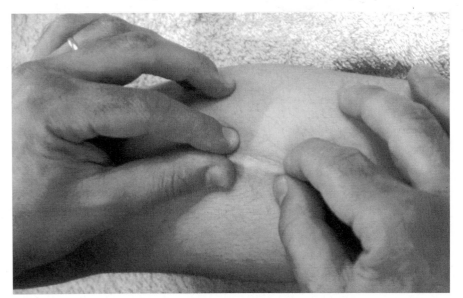

Figure 69
Longitudinal Tension Test
of a Scar

Of course, we only normalize the lesion of the dermis if it is a primary or a dominant lesion. Our treatment will be done by recoil against the fascial barrier, and we should notice that immediately the cutaneous layer returns to its normal elasticity and gliding in relation to the subjacent tissue.

After the adjustment, the skin roll allows us to verify that the skin has regained its normal flexibility and is pain free. If there is cellulite in this area, we should visibly notice that the thickness, as well as the volume, has decreased.

For the special case of cutaneous scarring, we do a specific test of longitudinal traction, as if we want to close the opening by stretching the scar at both ends. We remain quite superficial for this test, even for deeper scars from surgeries, because, in fact, improper closing at the cutaneous level disturbs the organism more than subjacent adhesions because it allows an *energetic leak*.

Another particular case is a point scar, a type we find more and more due to arthroscopic surgeries or drains. We mobilize it in all four directions, and especially clockwise and counterclockwise, to find the point of maximal retraction upon which we must act.

If we find a fixation of the scar in these cases, we will balance it with any other lesions of the cutaneous

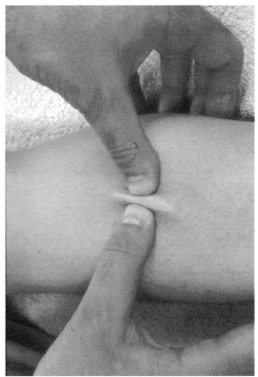

Figure 70
Transverse Pressure Test of a Scar

system in order to determine the dominant lesion of the dermis.

The cutaneous dominant lesion will be balanced with the ones of the other functional units to determine the primary lesion of the entire osteopathic entity. If we have to treat a scar as a primary or a dominant lesion, we will adjust it by means of longitudinal stretching (recoil).

The Treatment

Due to the many important functions of the skin, it seems impossible to ignore this 1.5 square meters of connective tissue that surrounds the body. However, it is not practical to treat all the cutaneous zones or scars that we find, and not only that, but they are often reflexive, and therefore secondary. In practice, we notice that the lesions of the dermis are qualitative rather than quantitative: if they "survive" in the inhibitory balancing test, they end up being the second or the third dominant. Thus, in Mechanical Link, we neither neglect or privilege work on the skin, but logically and coherently integrate it into the general evaluation. As a final intervention within the global context of a well-conducted treatment, work with the dermis presents a finishing touch.

15

Modalities and Particular Perspectives

This chapter presents some particular applications of Mechanical Link's approach and methods.

The Directed Treatment

We have developed a shorter Mechanical Link protocol for quickly determining treatment priority, i.e. the focus likely to result in the most nociceptive effect on the function of the organism.

Osteopathy, chiropractic, and other manual therapies emphasize the spine. Our *directed treatment*, while not limiting the treatment to the spine, will use the spine as the diagnostic axis for evaluation. In fact, the segmental constitution of the human being takes its organization from the spine, and a significant pathological tissular lesion anywhere in the body will tend to facilitate the corresponding vertebral segment. This connection of a particular vertebral level with its segmental territory supports the reality of the mechanical and the neurology link that unify them.

We start the directed treatment with the evaluation of the occipito-vertebral-pelvic axis as we have presented it (in Chapter 7). Once we are done, we will have found the dominant lesion of the spine, the lesion that we consider the key to one or more fixations situated in the segmental territory of this vertebral level. We then focus the rest of our evaluation on all articular, osseous, visceral, vascular, and cutaneous structures in direct relation with the dominant lesion of the occipito-vertebral-pelvic axis. Following our usual tension tests, we will find the fixations present in these territories. We must then balance the different lesions against one another to find the dominant one and then compare the *peripheral* lesion in relation to the *central* lesion of the vertebral axis, which will give us the dominant lesion of this somite.

The treatment will obviously start with the adjustment of this dominant lesion, whether it is in the vertebral area or in the corresponding peripheral territory. After the normalization of this dominant lesion and verification of the secondary lesions that may persist, we will neutralize the dominant vertebral lesion. We will then check all the other lesions of the occipito-vertebral-pelvic axis that we had previously found. If one or more lesions of the spine remain, we must then treat the peripheral segmental territory of the next most dominant lesion.

At the end of this directed treatment, because we have neutralized all of the central (vertebral) and peripheral (situated at a distance) lesions that were nociceptive enough to create a vertebral imbalance, we should end up with the normalization of the whole occipito-vertebral-pelvic axis.

The vertebral system is similar to a keyboard console: all excessive hypertension no matter where it is located, will show as a lesion on the vertebral system corresponding to the mechanical or neurological level responsible. By using the vertebral system as a console our treatment protocol allows us to focus on the essential, i.e. towards the most significant osteopathic lesion of the vertebral system.

The directed treatment is not symptomatic because no matter what the patient's complaint the focus will be on evaluation of the vertebral system to diagnose the biomechanical disturbances responsible. The directed treatment is not as complete as the general treatment but it is faster, brings about global balance, and gives us good clinical results, which encourages us to continue our research in that direction.

Targeting

We call *targeting* any deliberate intervention on a biomechanical unit that the global test does not show to have a significant lesion. Targeting systematically acts on the lesional parameters of an individual unit that suffers. It allows normalizing the minor lesions of an individual unit that was not strong enough to create a positive global test, but that was participating in the symptoms of a particular area. Targeting is not only done on the osteoarticular or visceral structures that have to be treated but also on the intraosseous lines of force, the arteries, and the dermis in relation to the concerned territory.

First we do all the specific tests of the unit to be treated, and then we do the inhibitory balancing tests to find the dominant lesion(s) implicated. Then we carry out adjustment with the recoil, limiting this to the second phase (see Chapter 6) in order to deliberately reduce the reach of the intervention to this level.

Targeting is to the general treatment what the tactics are to the strategy in the military; it is a commando action that will achieve a designated objective. *We use targeting mainly in two cases: for emergencies and for persistent localized symptoms.*

Emergencies

We talk about osteopathic emergencies only if three conditions are present together:
- *acute affliction*, i.e. any crisis that needs quick intervention;
- *recent affliction*, i.e. symptoms that have started less than a week ago and that are not a recurring problem;
- *functional affliction*, excluding all severe pathologies that would fall into the medical or surgical domain.

In cases of emergency, the focus of the treatment must be on the implicated functional unit(s). Our first intention is to neutralize the dominant lesion(s) of these functional units and then to target the afflicted individual unit. For example, for acute sinusitis, we first examine the cephalic unit in detail to diagnose and treat the dominant lesion(s), then, symptomatically adjust all the minor lesions that locally participate in the sinusitis. For lumbago, we test the spine and the lower extremities in order to act on the dominant of the two functional units. Once this has been done, we can target the lumbar vertebrae and the pelvis.

Of course, the treatment in case of emergency is not as complete and elaborate as the normal evaluation and treatment, but when necessary, it allows us to act very quickly to address the reason for the consultation and to quickly release a lot of acute afflictions such as torticollis, articular sprain, asthma attack, migraine, painful menses, acute hemorrhoids, neuralgia, and so on.

Due to the simplicity of application, the targeting treatment for emergencies can be done in any situation or location (office, home, sports field, etc.).

Persistent Symptoms

Symptoms sometimes persist after two or three visits during which a general treatment was done, that is, there is little or no improvement of the condition that the patient consulted us for. In this case, even if the global test does not objectively show a significant local restriction, we must target the territory that is suffering.

For instance, Mr. R.D., fifty-years old, consulted us for arthritis of the right shoulder, resistant to all previous treatment (anti-inflammatory medications, injections, and physiotherapy). He had been in pain without any release for over two years. After two visits, Mr. R.D. felt much better overall, and his digestion and his sleep had improved. However, although there was a bit more range of motion at the right shoulder, he continued to have as much pain as ever, especially at night. During the first two visits we had not intervened on the right shoulder because the global test of the shoulder girdle was negative. On the third visit, after the global treatment, we decided to act symptomatically on the minor lesions that were present in the right shoulder girdle. Mr. R.D. called us three weeks later to tell us that the pain had greatly decreased. When he returned four months later for a consolidating treatment, he told us that he did not feel any pain at all in his shoulder.

As this case shows, targeting has a place within the overall global treatment, allowing us to intervene locally to address the symptoms that brought people in for treatment and to assist in the overall healing process.

Bombarding

Bombarding is a variation of targeting that allows us to adjust all the minor restrictions of an individual functional unit within the context of addressing symptoms. It differs from targeting, in which the lesions are first related to one another in hierarchy so that only the dominant ones are treated. In bombarding we treat all the lesions as soon as we find them during the specific tests.

The adjustments are done using phase one of the recoil so that our action stays quite localized.

Out intent is a bit like that of "meta-therapy": we are looking to intervene on many points in the zone of discomfort; whereas, targeting acts more precisely like an injection would. Bombarding is to targeting what the burst of a machine gun is to a shot from a precision rifle. In the same way, the goal of bombarding is not to hit one specific point but to bombard every lesion in the territory by treating each as we find it.

Bombarding may be done with the patient in a neutral position or in a position that increases the symptoms. We can then adjust a meniscal blockage in the flexion position of the knee that is the most stuck. We can bombard a vertebral segment in the position of the spine that increases the pain or normalize a temporomandibular joint either with the mouth open to increase to range of motion, or with the mouth closed to balance an occlusion.

In practice, bombarding allows the practitioner to adapt to all situations and to give a symptomatic response to a local affliction.

Working with Pregnant Women

To avoid or to minimize the inherent disturbances during pregnancy, it is recommended to treat pregnant women during all the different phases of gestation. From the first to the third month, the consultation follows the same protocol as a regular visit, but avoids any too direct work in the gynecological sphere. From the third to the eighth month the modification of the gravid uterus calls for particular attention to the pelvic area.

In functional anatomy, the gravid uterus may be considered like a typical muscle with its various components:
- The body of the uterus is similar to the muscle belly.
- The inferior segment, the lower and narrow part of the uterus is similar to the tendon of the uterine muscle.

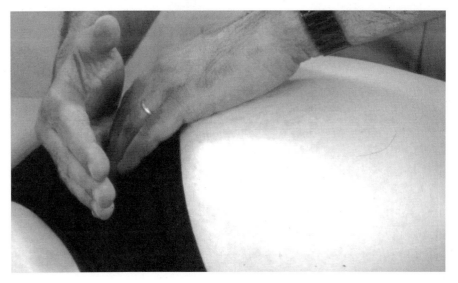

Figure 71

Tension Test of the Inferior Part of the Gravid Uterus (Patient Supine)

- The cervix, fixated and varying very little in size during the pregnancy, is similar to the insertion of the uterine muscle.
- The segmental fascia that covers the uterus and that sticks closely to the myometrium corresponds to the aponeurosis of the uterine muscle.

After our global balancing treatment, it is then interesting to specifically test the uterus in all three dimensions and to assess the tonicity of its wall. All fixations of the uterus will lead to the usual complications of pregnancy (uterine contractions, lumbago, hemorrhoids, etc.) that a well-placed targeting intervention at this level can treat or prevent.

The lesions that we encounter the most are right side-bending of the uterus, right torsion, and lower fixation of the uterus. The right side-bending, because it tends to compress the inferior vena cava, often leads to swollen legs, varicose veins, cardiac palpitations, and to all vascular troubles that seem to be aggravated lying down. The right torsion of the uterus leads to lumbago or sciatica. The lowered position of the uterus leads to uterine contractions and also to the risk of miscarriages or to premature labor.

Besides the uterus, we must also target other areas:
- the dermis of the abdomen to prevent stretch marks;
- the lines of force of the pubis and the axis of the sacrum to stabilize the pelvis;

Figure 72

Rotation Test of the Body of the Uterus (Patient Sitting Up)

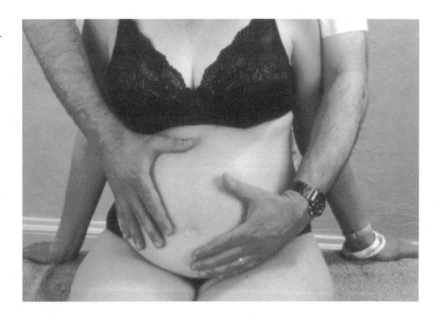

- the vascular system of the lower extremities to decrease circulatory problems;
- the thoracic diaphragm and the superior stomach to prevent acid reflux.

In the ninth month, the consultation goes over all the points that we have previously examined, but we also concentrate on preparation for labor and delivery. In general, even though our treatment must remain light during the pregnancy, at full term we can put more intensity into our work. In the preparation for labor, we must bombard all the restrictions, even the minor ones that may affect the uterus or the pelvic girdle, including the coccyx.

At times we might be called upon to work on breach presentation. Unlike the obstetrical maneuvers that try to more or less force the fetus to turn, we simply normalize the clockwise and counterclockwise rotation that is always present in the gravid uterus. We have obtained many "spontaneous" turnings of the fetus in the few days following the treatment, or even if the fetus didn't turn, delivery was easier.

Working with Infants

Many qualified osteopaths have written on this subject, and we only want here to add few clinical observations. With Mechanical Link, we do a global osteopathic evaluation for an infant the same way as we do for an adult—aiming to find the primary lesion, without any special attention paid to the cranium or to any other functional unit. Even if certain lesions, for example, those of the ossification centers on the cranium, the thoracic esophagus, the head of the pancreas, or the intraosseous bowing of the tibia, are statistically more common in the infant, we must systematically test a baby as completely as we do an adult, without any preconceived ideas.

We observe the posture of the infant by suspending him or her in the air, holding him or her under the arms. Most often, the baby shows a "comma-like" inclination of the spine, with a lateral translation of the pelvis at times. The degree of inclination is in proportion to the severity of the fascial tension that is present. After this observation, we can add the palpation of the shape of the cranial vault, noticing the roundness or the flat areas, which gives us information on the postural schematic of the osseous head. The results of the observation and of the palpation may be observed by the parents. After the treatments, the visible improvement of the posture or of the shape of the head is a better witness to what we can do for their child than any speech we can give them.

We test the spine of the infant with him or her lying flat on the stomach or in the arms of the parents. The examination of the extremities is preferably done using traction. The examination of the viscera is more succinct than with adults and must take into consideration the anatomical differences such as the larger liver and thymus in the baby.

Generally, the tension tests that we use on the newborn are the same as the ones we use for the adult. The recoil will also be identical except that we will remain in phase two because the baby cannot voluntarily participate in respiration. Since lesions in newborns are not very long-standing, they react very well to our treatment, and we usually have good results with one or two visits.

The Anti-Tobacco Treatment

Mechanical Link is a type of global manual therapy that allows us to approach diverse health issues, and the anti-tobacco treatment is one more possibility in this arsenal of functional medicine.

In practice, we ask a patient to completely stop the use of tobacco forty-eight hours before the treatment. This abrupt and total withdrawal creates a metabolic and psychological stress, a crisis situation that we then approach following our usual protocol. The general examination will show particular lesions that are not only related to the usual diathesis of the patient but also related to the acute withdrawal from tobacco.

This approach to the problem focuses on both circumstances and structure, and it is interesting for several reasons:

- It does not obviate the individual making a decision to stop smoking, and in fact it helps in the process.
- It allows for a treatment that is adapted to the individual because the lesions found during the evaluation will vary from one patient to the next.
- It is not palliative but regulatory because it helps the organism itself to find physiological equilibrium.

We have now used this Mechanical Link approach with about fifty people, including some who had tried different techniques without success. We were able to help about eighty percent completely give up use of tobacco. We hope that this treatment protocol will be expanded through its use by the different practitioners of Mechanical Link. Moreover, we hope that the therapists that work in relation with drug and alcohol abuse will also be able to introduce Mechanical Link as an added method and share their results.

Working with Animals

While treating a few dogs and horses with Mechanical Link, we observed that the body structure of animals responds well to the tension test, the inhibitory balancing test, and to the recoil technique. A few techniques must be adapted; for example, testing a horse often requires two persons to do the inhibitory balancing because two lesions may be too far from one another for one practitioner to reach.

It may be that the Mechanical Link approach will expose some lesions that are little known in veterinary osteopathy. For example, we were surprised to find lesions in a horse's hoof.

Many Mechanical Link practitioners that work in the equine world report interesting results; we hope that they will share their experiences.

Treatment and Self-Treatment of the Fascial Link

In most cases Mechanical Link can be used as a self-treatment. This represents a small revolution in the classical practice of osteopathy in which the patient's treatment is in the hands and under the direction of the practitioner. And yet, there have been many times when a colleague was not available to treat us, and so we have worked on ourselves. Little by little we have established a protocol of self-treatment based on the tension tests and the recoil adjustment. We have called this protocol the *treatment and self-treatment of the fascial link* (TSFL). The TSFL can be used by the practitioner on the patient (treatment) or on him or her self (self-treatment).

As its name indicates, the TSFL is a form of treatment and self-treatment that harmonizes the diverse tissular structures of the organism in a logical manner. Through experience, we have chosen to work with three functional units that cover the total body: the intraosseous lines of force, the arteries, and the derma.

For the self-treatment, one needs to be lying down or seated comfortably. From this position, we perform (on our own body) a series of tests of the structure to be treated. This self-treatment repeats the protocol of the tension test, except that in self-treatment the lesions are adjusted as soon as we find them.

We proceed in this fashion from the deepest to most superficial, by releasing our osseous, vascular, and cutaneous structures. Once we have treated the lesions of these three systems, we can also act on any specific territory (e.g. the osseous head, the visceral unit, the articular system of the extremities, etc.). If we want to treat a particular function or symptom, we do so using the recoil phase one or two.

Self-treatment is recommended once or twice a week to maintain a good rhythm and in order to expand the effect of the TSFL treatment. The positive effect of the TSFL is felt immediately: it increases general flexibility of the body, thoracic expansion, energy, intellectual stimulation, general relaxation, etc. The TSFL is useful in preparing for a sporting event, and participants in certain activities (e.g. aikido, yoga, and qi-gong) have reported an increased perception of the circulation of energy.

The TSFL is not a substitute for the therapeutic effects of treatment based on the diagnosis of the total lesion (by placing lesions in a hierarchy) but allows for a general stimulation of the most important functions of the organism. We know that the structure/function relationship is reciprocal: the integrity of the structure conditions its activities (according to Still, the structure governs the function); and also physiological activity is necessary for the existence of the structure (according to Pavlov, the function creates the organ).

Osteopathy tries to normalize the biomechanics of the body's structures in order to improve its function. The TSFL stimulates and maintains the state of our organism in order to improve the structure. Man is born a soft being and dies a hard one. This inevitable process of tissular aging reflects the pathway of all pathologies, which tend to start in the realm of function and progressively evolve towards an increasingly irreversible change of the structure. From this we can see the importance of harmonizing that complementary pair: structure and function. The TSFL does not replace osteopathic treatment but is complementary and true to the spirit of Mechanical Link.

A general knowledge of osteopathy is necessary for a good application of the TSFL, and only practitioners that have been trained in Mechanical Link should apply the TSFL. We are especially concerned about working with the arteries—delicate and complex structures that require perfect manual mastery of the technique in order to safely apply it. However, because the TSFL increases the general flexibility of the body, activates fluid circulation, and stimulates certain physiological functions of the organism, it is a powerful aid to practitioners of Mechanical Link for managing and maintaining their own health.

16

The Energetic Approach

Mechanical or Energetic Vision?

O steopathy is considered *functional medicine*, based on the principle that a vital force drives the organism and, normally, maintains its health.

Certain therapeutic approaches, such as homeopathy or traditional Chinese medicine, to name just a couple, are based on a highly developed understanding of the energetic function of the organism. However, osteopathy seems to still be looking for its identity, not sure whether to take an orthopedic or manipulative direction or to adopt a fluid, global, and subtle approach. In Mechanical Link we privilege neither the more mechanical structural techniques nor the more functional energetic techniques but rather suggest a third path that links those two complementary aspects of osteopathy.

The Concept of Energy in Osteopathy

Some approaches to health try to integrate the notion of energy into manual practice by making use of certain subtle manifestations of the organism using iridology, pulse diagnosis (traditional Chinese medicine), kineseology, spectography, etc. Although these methods objectively diagnose energetic phenomenon, they are less direct approaches. Osteopathy operates on the basis of a much more direct reading of energetic reality. Energy is matter in movement ($E=mc^2$), and our science is based upon this concept. The osteopath directly identifies the restriction of mobility (movement) of the structure (matter), i.e. the decrease of the energetic potential due to the tissular fixation that affects it.

Sources of Errors in Different Approaches

We will describe the principle in order to be clear: if a patient is observed to have a positive hepatic iris sign, a tense pulse, a thermal zone, or a positive kineseology test in relation to the right side of abdomen, this would be taken as a manifestation of an energetic disturbance of the liver, while osteopathic testing might not demonstrate any fixation of this organ. In our view, the primary or dominant lesion that causes restriction of mobility or hepatic malfunction may be located elsewhere in the body, and that is where we should act and not on the liver itself.

If we give an osteopathic treatment to an element that was located by other criteria than the mobility tests, we always risk acting wrongly. Thus, we are convinced that osteopathy has its own means of palpatory investigation, and therefore of energetic diagnosis. Manual treatment should be applied exclusively in response to the results of the mobility tests. Osteopathy is complete on its own!

We must always keep in mind the gap that exists between the nature of the osteopathic lesion and the energetic manifestations that it brings. In the thermal approach, for example, restriction of mobility is thought to correspond to a cold or hot zone. However, we believe that the phase it is in affects the temperature, that is, during the inflammatory or spasmodic phase we associate tissular hyperactivity with heat, whereas a slowing down of the metabolism and decrease in temperature accompanies the fibrotic and the sclerotic phases. Even if temporary reactivity occurs during the fibrotic phase, there is no correlation between the thermal zone and the restriction of mobility that may be found due to the fascial tension. In osteopathy, we must consider the structural causes and not the effects that result from it (heat, pain, modification of the pulses, or any other energetic manifestations).

We suppose that even the original practitioners of acupuncture must have had a direct palpatory perception of the points to be treated. Based on that, they must have developed an intellectual model for understanding and teaching the following generations. But behind the complex coded systems that inform us, we can find a simple and direct knowledge of things, one that no amount of reasoning, as intelligent as it might be, can ever give us.

Still's aphorism—*find it, fix it, leave it alone*—must be exactly followed, as it constitutes the original foundation for a mechanical as well as an energetic approach to health.

The Different Energetic Territories

Experience has showed us that not all anatomical units represent the same nature and potential of energy.

- The spinal keyboard gives an autonomic response that is quite strong and rapid but that is relatively segmental.
- The articulations of the extremities, especially of the lower extremities, have a great energetic capacity, and this quantitative contribution is often critical for the organism to recharge itself.
- The value of the visceral system, usually less implicated in the primary lesion, has a more subtle and qualitative nature.
- The intraosseous lines of force, to which the acupuncture meridians have some correspondence, are an important energetic reserve that, once released, will deeply revitalize most of the vital functions but need time to fully develop.
- The circulating and immediately available energy of the vascular system has a quick manifestation of its effects.
- The thorax, more specifically the anterior aspect, relates to the energetic rhythm and to certain emotional phenomena.
- The osseous head, more complex in its details, presents different global characteristics, depending on which floor: inferior (instinctive functions), middle (sensorial functions) and superior (cerebral functions).
- The derma—the unit that is the least biomechanically structured—corresponds more to the surface energy, and relates to the external environment, expressing only superficially the disturbances underneath. We can talk of the *cutaneous interface.*

We prefer not to detail more of the many energetic correspondences that we have noticed—it would be an extensive list! Such statements as that the anterior attachment of the falx cerebri corresponds to insomnia, even if statistically accurate, would lead to false assumptions, e.g. for insomnia treat the falx cerebri. We assert most strongly that such "recipes" are not efficient because they are symptomatic, and so, not osteopathic! Thus, in our example, if the fascial restriction on the falx cerebri is dependant on another lesion, it is this latter one—the one that is dominant—and not the previous one, that is secondary, that we must act upon in order to have an improvement of sleeping. We also wish to avoid a misleading synthesis of approach. Even if our observations in relation to the energetic system correspond to the observations of those in other types of functional medicine, the coherence and the specificity of each approach must be respected.

Modifications in Osteopathic Lesion Patterns and Energetic Rhythms

Living things constantly evolve, and the patterns of restriction of mobility that make up the total lesion are not a fixed and immovable schematic. The intensity of blockages varies and is modulated, depending on the different activities of the organism, the external context, the proper biorhythm, and other factors. The organization of the lesional schematic constantly modifies itself in a sensible fashion.

For example, if T–9 is the primary lesion of a specific patient at a specific time, it is possible that at a different time of day or after a sporting activity, the lesion at T–9, without disappearing, may be of a lesser intensity and not primary but under the influence of another lesion. Therefore, it is very important that the treatment adapts to the exact need of the organism, right here, right now, during the consultation.

Is it really necessary to study the different hourly, daily, lunar, menstrual, seasonal—energetic rhythms—to take into consideration the gender, the profession, the constitution of the patient or other parameters that in practice are hard to reconcile totally? Thankfully, no! Nature gives a simple answer when we ask the right question. The osteopath only needs to systematically evaluate the structure, and the structure—the foundation and underpinning of homeostasis—will reveal the true energetic needs of the organism with clarity and intelligence.

The Energetic Approach of Mechanical Link

A qualified practitioner nowadays has many different techniques to normalize a restriction of mobility, but our personal preference will always be the recoil; this technique of correction combines the mechanical and the energetic aspects of osteopathy.

The mechanical aspect is necessary because diastases, articular subluxation, disc compression, or restriction in an intraosseous line of force will not be corrected just by blowing on them. However, the energetic aspect is also necessary because the head of the pancreas, an osteoporotic vertebra, a gravid uterus, a nonconsolidated fracture, an abdominal heart, or an artery are not manipulated by "hammering" on them.

In practice, the recoil adapts easily to the exact degree of the fascial barrier and allows release of any element of the body without force. The recoil restores the organism's ability to move, and therefore, restores its energetic potential, without risking trauma or destabilizing the structure.

In the formula $E=mc^2$ the speed (squared) is greater than the mass; this explains why the impact of the recoil is so great. The dynamic of the movement requires extreme speed of impulsion, but the physical push or force behind the maneuver remains small (much less than that in classical manipulations). Thus, the energy released is great. The recoil combines the vigor of structural techniques with the gentleness of functional techniques.

The Recoil Technique and Energetic Action

The variations in use of the recoil allow the energetic action of our adjustment to be modulated to suit our requirements. The objective of phase two is to look for the maximal point of tension of the fascial barrier (phase one) and then to explore the three dimensions in space. The horizontal and the vertical sweep allow the adjustment to be precise in its mechanical spatial dimension, whereas the parameters of clockwise and counterclockwise rotation give more of an energetic twist to the recoil.

This aspect of energetic spiraling is found in acupuncture, created by the different maneuvers of the needle. (Experts in Chinese medicine do not agree about the proper directions for tonifying or dispersing the energy.) As for us, in practice we always follow what the structure indicates, i.e. by rotating in the direction of most tension, as if we wanted to screw in the tissues. This way it is not the practitioner that arbitrarily imposes the direction, but the wisdom of the structure that indicates its true need.

This fundamental notion that *only the tissues knows* is also what tells us the exact degree of rotation needed during the build up of tension; this degree will depend on the resistance felt by us, and we must stop precisely at the point of blockage that stops us (when the fascial barrier is felt like a notch that stops us from going farther).

In phases three and four of the recoil, which we have called *metabolic*, and where we for ask the active breathing of the patient, the accent is on the process of transformation of matter and energy by the organism itself. The respiration carries the breath of life, the rhythmic and harmonious alternation of inspiration and expiration, anabolism and catabolism, yin and yang, birth and death—and rebirth.

When the blockage on which we want to act hardens in the inhalation or the exhalation of the patient, it corresponds to an accumulation of tension of the osteopathic lesion with respiratory pressure. The apnea required for phase four will lock up the total lesion, and applying the recoil at that moment will revive the general metabolism of the organism. It is not a breathing exercise but a way to determine at which point the energetic rhythm of the osteopathic lesion has reached a peak of tension.

Respiration reveals and amplifies the blockage, and the other way around is also true: the neutralization of the blockage will be able to improve respiratory function. Classic osteopathy and other types of manual therapy often put a lot of emphasis on the fixations of the thoracic diaphragm in the lesional schematic. In the protocol of Mechanical Link, we systematically test this muscle at its center and both lateral leaflets; we have noticed that the restrictions of mobility here are most often secondary or adaptation lesions. The normalization of the primary or the dominant lesions will release the diaphragm and the respiration (and not the reverse!).

The exhalation is a relaxation period; however, it is interesting to notice that it is during this phase that osteopathic lesions tend to harden the most. This probably corresponds to the difficulty of our existential person to *let go*. When tension increases during the inhalation, the person has a problem with the anabolic functions: a difficulty assimilating, incorporating, and balancing the energy given to him or her.

In all cases, to obtain a full energetic balancing that is perfectly adapted to the particular patient we must treat each lesion individually and in the respiration phase that is indicated.

Osteopathy and Homeopathy

These two functional and energetic medicines that were developed at the same time in history and both in an occidental context, have different methods but some similarity in underlying approach.

In Mechanical Link, we systematically examine the subject, seeking to determine the pattern of lesions and arranging them in a hierarchy by means of the inhibitory balancing tests in order to find out and treat the dominant ones. We will decide which phase of the recoil is most appropriate depending on the type of fixation that needs to be treated, and, after the normalization, we will let the healing force of the organism act as necessary.

In classical homeopathy, the practitioner will methodically interview the patient, bring to light all the symptoms, and then assign values to the symptoms in order to find and work with the most important ones. He or she will choose the most appropriate dilution-dynamisation for the type of pathology to be treated, and after the medication has been taken, will let the therapeutic capacities of the organism come into play to bring about healing.

However, even though similarities in the fundamental principles and the protocol for treatment are evident, the two forms of medicine do not operate at the same level: the osteopathic treatment intervenes mostly on the energetic foundation (the structure, the *memory of the bone*); whereas, the homeopathic treatment acts on the nature of the energy (the substance, the *memory of the water*). Therefore, they are complementary, and a therapeutic synergy benefits a lot of patients.

Osteopathy and Acupuncture

Acupuncture, which represents only one branch of Chinese medicine, is practiced too often outside of its geographical, cultural, and therapeutic context. Many osteopaths who have taken some training in this area integrate the use of needles into their treatments; however, we think this brings confusion in both principles and practice.

Unlike homeopathy, acupuncture intervenes at almost the same level as osteopathy, because it proposes to address the circulation of energy by using key points of the structure. Thus we observe that acupuncture and osteopathy are not *complementary*, and that using them together represents too much of a good thing. We run the risk of interference and of saturation of information when both treatments are used within a short time span, or even worse, if they are used in the same visit.

We have noticed that successfully combining treatment with osteopathy and treatment with acupuncture or ear acupuncture requires allowing enough time between sessions. We must also note that more people are developing an aversion to the use of needles and or to manipulation. We must be aware of these attitudes and respect them, so as to be at the service of our patients.

The Structure as an Energetic Support

Osteopathy has the means to concretely approach the subtle manifestation of energy via the structure. We must use the intelligence and the logic of the structure as the basis for our treatment—to let it be at the same time the support of our action, our guide, and our reference. If structure governs function, it is because homeostasis depends upon the condition of the structure. For an etiological and global treatment of the structure, we must take into consideration all mechanical and energetic aspects of the total lesion. With Mechanical Link, we propose a rational method to efficiently help the organism to find again its physical equilibrium and the energetic potential necessary for good health.

CHAPTER 17

Conclusion

The hand is a marvelous therapeutic tool for the one who takes the time and the effort to educate it with great discipline. In this spirit, Mechanical Link gives practitioners a simple, efficient, and logical way to practice this art.

The tension tests allow us to examine the whole body with simplicity and to discover all of the existing lesions. The balance tests allow us to logically order those lesions into a hierarchy so as to find the dominant and the primary lesions. The recoil allows us to efficiently adjust the dominant and the primary lesions in order to directly or indirectly normalize all the existing lesions.

Using the specific techniques of the Mechanical Link, we have been able to explore new anatomical areas that until now had been neglected, misunderstood, or difficult to approach. Some of our discoveries include working with articular diastasis, fixation of the intraosseous lines of force, or lesions of the arteries, all of which play a considerable role in the pathology in many cases. To know how to evaluate and to treat lesions in these areas represents great progress for manual therapy. However, in spite of the excellence of our results, Mechanical Link assigns a modest role to the practitioner, who should intervene as little as possible and must have confidence in nature. (As A.T. Still said, "Find it; fix it; leave it alone.")

Even if the rigor of our protocols may give the opposite impression, Mechanical Link is not a rigid and closed system. The objectivity and the reproducibility of the tests make Mechanical Link a heuristic: open to change and also possibly helpful as a model for practitioners of other systems. We have a lot of respect and admiration for our many colleagues that actively participate, some brilliantly, in the evolution of manual therapies. We hope that the work of us all will create in this new millennium a more human, more ecological, more authentic medicine.

Bibliography

Agur, Anne M.R. and Ming J. Lee. *Grant's Atlas of Anatomy*. Philadelphia: Williams & Wilkins, 1999.

Barral, Jean-Pierre. *Trauma: An Osteopathic Approach*. Seattle: Eastland Press, 1999.

Barral, Jean-Pierre and Pierre Mercer. *Visceral Manipulation*. Seattle: Eastland Press, 1988.

Barral, Jean-Pierre, *Visceral Manipulation II*. Seattle: Eastland Press, 1989.

Chauffour, Paul and Jean-Marle Guillot. *Le Lien Mechanique Osteopathique*. Paris: Maloine, 1985.

Chauffour, Paul and Ange Castejon. *Techniques Peripheriques*. n.p.: Ed Osteopathic Management Company, n.d.

Clemente, Carmine D. *Anatomy: A Regional Atlas of the Human Body*. Baltimore: Williams & Wilkins, 1997.

Kahle, W., H. Leonhardt, W. Platzer, and C. Cabrol (dir.). *Anatomie 2: Visceres*. Paris: Flammarion Medecine-Science, 1980.

Kamina, Pierre. *Dictionaire Atlas d'Anatomie*. Paris: Maloine, 1999.

Moore, Keith L. and T.V.N. Persaud. *The Developing Human: Clinically Oriented Embryology*. Philadelphia: Saunders, 1998.

Netter, Frank H., *Atlas of Human Anatomy*. East Hanover: Novartis, 1997.

Paoletti, Serge. *Les Fascias*. Vannes Cedex: Sully, 1998.

Perronneaud-Ferre, R. *Techniques Reflexes En Osteopathie*. Aix en Provence: Verlague, 1999.

Piganiol, G. *Les Manipulations Vertebrales*. Aix en Provence: Verlague, n.d.

Still, A.T. *Osteopathy: Research and Practice*. Seattle: Eastland Press, 1992.

Tortora, Gerard J. and Nicholas Anagnostakos. *Principles of Anatomy & Physiology*. New York: Harper & Row, 1987.

Upledger, John E. *A Brain is Born*. Berkeley: North Atlantic Books, 1996.

Venes, Donald (editor). *Taber's Cyclopedic Medical Dictionary*. Philadelphia: F.A. Davis Co, 1993.

Voll, Reinhold, *Topographic Positions of the Measurement Points in Electro-Acupuncture*. Velzen: Medizinisch Lieterarische Verlagsgesellschaft, 1976.

Zilbermann, S. *Architecture Cranio-Sacree*. Aix en Provence: Verlague, 2000.

Index

Fasciae
    anterior vs. posterior, 10
    deep, 15–19
    different systems of, 9
    dura mater, 19–21
    latae, 14
    superficial, 10–15
    superficialis, 21–22
Feet, 80, 92. *See also* Extremities
Fibrosis, 24–25, 149
Fryman, V., 131
Fundus, 106

G
Gall bladder, 107–8
Genital sphere, 111–13
Global respiratory movement, 50
Global tests, 37. *See also individual functional units*
Goetz, E. W., 101
Golgi, receptors of, 53

H
Hands, 78, 93. *See also* Extremities
Head. *See* Cephalic unit (osseous head)
Heart
    embryological development of, 4, 7
    fixations of, 119–20
    testing, 117–18
    vascular system and, 126
Herniated disk, 64–65
Hips, 79
Homeopathy, 25, 165, 170–71
Horses, working with, 161
Hyoid bone, 11
Hypermobility, 84

I
Ileum, 66–67, 109–10
Iliac crest, 59–60
Iliac fascia, 13
Infants, working with, 159–60

Infections, 26–27
Inflammation, 24, 25, 149
Inguinal ligament, 13, 110
Inhalation, 48–49, 170
Inhibitory balancing test, 38–40
Injured tissue, 24
Intestines
    large, 109
    small, 108
Intraosseous lines of force, 87–99
    calcification and, 90
    of the cephalic unit, 94–95, 145–46
    cranial ossification centers and, 98
    examination and treatment protocol for, 97
    external, intermediary, and internal, 88
    fixated, 90
    of the iliac crest, 59–60
    importance of, 98–99
    working with, 91–97

K
Kidneys
    embryological development of, 8
    testing, 113–14
    vascular system and, 126–27
Knees, 79–80

L
Lambda, 144
Large intestine, 109
Larynx, 115
Legs. *See* Extremities
Lesions, 23–30. *See also* Recoil technique; *individual functional units*
    breathing and, 48–49
    causes of, 26–27
    definition of, 23, 87
    determination of, 35–36
    of diastasis, 65–66, 82–84
    first or original, 29
    genesis of, 24–26

individual, 27–28
modifications in patterns of, 168
primary, 28–30, 40, 42, 75
total, 9, 28, 38
Ligaments
inguinal, 13, 110
of Treitz, 18
Lines of force. *See* Intraosseous lines of force
Littlejohn, John Martin, xxiii
Liver, 114–15
Long bones, lesions of, 80–82
Lumbar fascia, 13
Lungs, 115

M

Magoun, H. I., 131
Mandible, 139–40
Mastoid, 139, 142
Mechanical Link. *See also* Recoil technique; *individual functional units*
anatomical view of, 8
balancing system and, 38
benefits of, 173
characteristics of, xxi–xxii
energetic approach of, 168–69
openness of, 173–74
role of practitioner in, 173
Mediastinum, 17
Mentalization, 50–51, 52
Mesenchyme, 3, 8
Mesoblast
cardiovascular system and, 7–8
diagram of, 2
as a link, 1–2
myofascial system and, 4–5
osseous system and, 5–7
Mesoderm, 2, 87
Muscles
arteries and, 124
embryological development of, 4
Myofascial system, 4–5

N

Nasal fossa, 142
Necrosis, 25
Nervous system
autonomic, 125–26
peripheral, 125

O

Obturator membrane, 110
Occiput, 57
Orbits, 143
Orthotics, 34
Osseous head. *See* Cephalic unit
Osseous system
architectural model of, 89–90
embryological development of, 5–7
functions of, 90–91
Ossification, membranous vs. endochondral, 5
Osteopathic lesions. *See* Lesions
Osteopathy
acupuncture and, 171
American vs. European branches of, xxiii–xxiv
classical focus of, 87
concept of energy in, 165–66, 172
as functional medicine, 165
history of, xxiii–xxiv
holistic vision of, 28
homeopathy and, 170–71
techniques in, 43–44

P

Pacini, receptors of, 53
Palate, hard, 141
Pancreas, 114
Paranasal sinuses, 142–43
Pelvic diaphragm, 111
Pelvis, 58–59, 96, 109–11
Pericardium, 117–18
Peripheral nervous system, 125
Peritoneum, 4
Pharynx, 105
Pia mater, 5

About the Authors

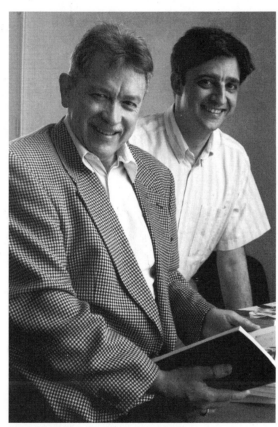

Paul Chauffour (left) and Eric Prat

PAUL CHAUFFOUR, D.O., is one of the most influential and renowned osteopaths in Europe and a pioneer in the field of Mechanical Link. He has authored two books, *Osteopathy of the Inferior Limbs* and *The Osteopathic Mechanical Link*. He teaches at the International College of Osteopathy in St. Etienne, France. In addition, he has taught at the European School of Osteopathy in Maidstone, England, and at the Faculty of Medicine in Paris North, Department of Osteopathy and Manual Medicine in Paris, France. He teaches Mechanical Link throughout the world.

ERIC PRAT, D.O., Major National 1987, has been practicing and teaching Mechanical Link since 1988 and is a protégé of Paul Chauffour's. He teaches at the A.T. Still Academy in Lyon and at the International College of Osteopathy in St. Etienne, France. He has teamed with the Upledger Institute to teach Mechanical Link seminars worldwide.

MONIQUE BUREAU, P.T., D.O., holds a Bachelor of Science degree in physical therapy from the University of Alberta, Edmonton, Canada, and a doctorate in osteopathic manual practice from the Canadian College of Osteopathy, Toronto, Canada. Bureau has practiced Mechanical Link in New York City since 1994. She teaches Mechanical Link courses throughout North America and has been Paul Chauffour's classroom translator for many years.